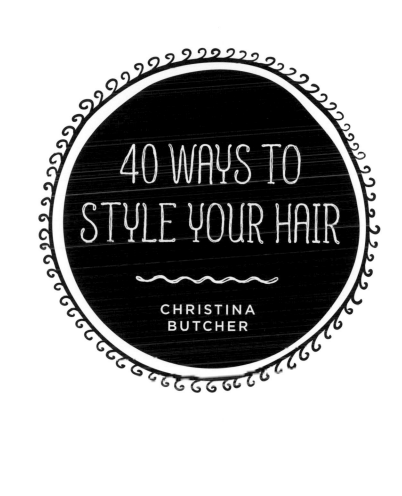

40 WAYS TO STYLE YOUR HAIR

CHRISTINA
BUTCHER

CHRONICLE BOOKS
SAN FRANCISCO

Published exclusively for Target in 2017 by Chronicle Books LLC.

Copyright © 2013 by RotoVision SA.

ISBN: 978-1-4521-5891-4

Library of Congress Cataloging-in-Publication Data available under the
original title, *Braids, Buns and Twists*, ISBN 978-1-4521-2484-1.

Manufactured in China.

Commissioning Editor: Isheeta Mustafi
Assistant Editor: Tamsin Richardson
Editor: Diane Leyman
Art Director: Emily Portnoi
Art Editor: Jennifer Osborne
Book layout: FentonForeman
Illustrations: Peters & Zabransky

10 9 8 7 6 5 4 3 2 1

Chronicle Books LLC
680 Second Street
San Francisco, CA 94107
www.chroniclebooks.com

This book is dedicated to Dad.
I miss you.

CONTENTS

PONYTAILS

BRAIDS

BUNS, KNOTS, AND TWISTS

BOUFFANTS

RESOURCES

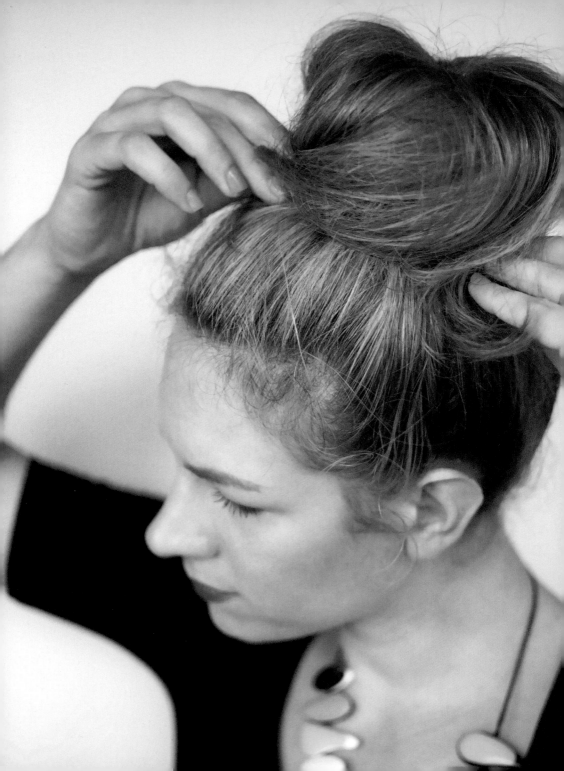

INTRODUCTION

Hello and welcome to *40 Ways to Style Your Hair*. This book puts all the tools at your disposal so that you'll never have another bad hair day. Ever!

Have you found yourself in the same hair rut, day in, day out? Have you had enough of wearing your hair the same way since . . . forever? Are you trying to grow out your hair, but looking for fun ways to wear it in the meantime? There's nothing worse than being in hair limbo, and that's where this book can help. There are enough styles and variations within these pages to give you a different hairstyle every day of the week for almost a quarter of the year—the only downside is that you might get tired of people asking how you did your hair!

This book guides you through each style so that you can make the most of your best accessory: your hair. Chapters are organized by broad hairstyle: Ponytails; Braids; Buns, Knots, and Twists; and Bouffants. Each hairstyle entry tells you what's involved and where the style comes from and offers examples for when and where it might work best. Each style is given a difficulty rating, and you'll find tips and ideas on how to vary the style and what accessories to try. A list of styling tools and easy-to-follow, illustrated step-by-step tutorials make creating the styles simple, and beautiful photography shows how these styles look and work in real life. At the back of the book you'll also find a resources chapter, which details hairstyling tools, schools and further education, and a glossary.

For me, discovering I could do so much with my hair really helped my confidence. I struggled for years to understand how to deal with it, and for a long time I hated it. Since learning how to treat my hair properly, I have finally come to love my hair. Now, when I see people trying out new styles in their own hair, I find it so inspiring.

40 Ways to Style Your Hair is here to help you practice and master all the techniques you need so that you can learn to love your hair too. This book shows how I create all my styles, and I know it won't be long before you love your hair just as much as I love mine. Your hair will become an exciting new part of your wardrobe that you can customize to go with whatever you're wearing and wherever you're going.

Enjoy the confidence your hair will bring. If I can do it, I know you can too!

QUIFFED PONYTAIL
THE LOOK

This ponytail is a fun hairstyle that transforms a plain pony into something special—it's a chic look but with just enough sass. To create this style, you'll tease the front and top of your hair to add height and volume. This style adds much needed length to a shorter face and has a fun retro feel.

DIFFICULTY LEVEL
Easy

IDEAL HAIR LENGTH
Long

HAIR EXTENSIONS NEEDED?
No, but you can use a ponytail extension on shorter hair.

ASSISTANCE NEEDED?
No

ACCESSORIES
The quiff acts as a kind of accessory so you don't need to add any more. A scarf or bow on the ponytail can add a retro twist.

TRY THIS
Experiment by combining this look with straight or curly hair. You can also twist the ponytail up into a bun to turn this great style into a cute updo.

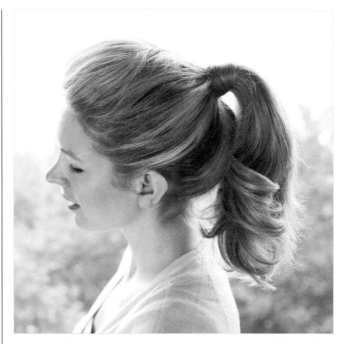

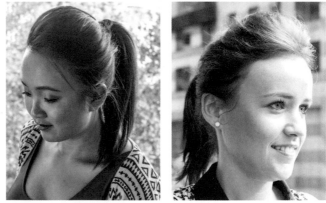

 SEE ALSO
Wrapped ponytail, pages 10–11
Gibson roll, pages 68–69

Top: Hairstyling and modeling by Christina Butcher, photography by Xiaohan Shen.
Bottom left: Hairstyling and photography by Christina Butcher, modeling by Adeline Er.
Bottom right: Hairstyling by Christina Butcher, photography by Xiaohan Shen, modeling by Sinead Brady.

HOW TO GET IT

WHAT YOU NEED

- Brush
- Teasing comb (optional)
- Bobby pins
- Hair elastic

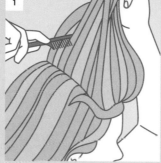

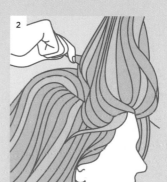

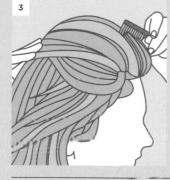

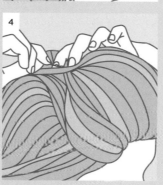

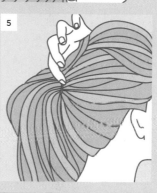

1–2. Lift the section of hair on the top of your head and begin backcombing your hair. Tease to create volume using a brush or teasing comb, starting at the crown and moving forward in sections toward your hairline.

3. Gently comb the top of your hair back over the teased quiff to smooth it and create the quiff shape.

4. Use a bobby pin just behind the quiff to secure it in place. Cross your bobby pins in an X shape for added hold.

5. Gather the rest of your hair up into a ponytail at the back of your head or place your ponytail a little higher, near your crown. Use an elastic to match your hair color, or wrap a small piece of hair around the elastic to hide it.

TOP TIP

If your hair is fine or soft, you'll need to use some product to hold the quiff and add volume. Before starting, apply mousse through your hair and blow-dry to add texture. You can also use hairspray to help hold the quiff in place, or use a sea salt product, which gives friction and helps to add volume.

WRAPPED PONYTAIL
THE LOOK

This wrapped ponytail is the perfect style if you have long hair and find it difficult to keep your ponytail in place. It is a casual yet sophisticated style that works from day to night. By leaving out the top section of hair, you'll find it easier to put the remainder of your hair up. You then wrap the top section around the base of the ponytail in a twisting motion. You angle your hair down as you wrap, and then your ponytail is pinned flat against the back of your head.

DIFFICULTY LEVEL
Medium

IDEAL HAIR LENGTH
Medium to long

HAIR EXTENSIONS NEEDED?
No, but you can use a ponytail extension on shorter hair.

ASSISTANCE NEEDED?
No

ACCESSORIES
Your hair is the accessory in this hairstyle, wrapping around your ponytail to create a twist. A jeweled clip or flower can be pinned into the side of the twist for a nighttime look.

TRY THIS
Adjust the position of the ponytail to give this hairstyle a different look. For instance, you could tie a really high ponytail or place it lower on the back of your head.

▶ **SEE ALSO**
Top knot bun, pages 64–65
French twist, pages 70–71

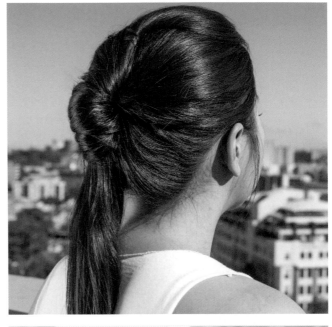

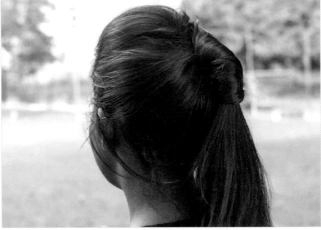

Top: Hairstyling and photography by Christina Butcher, modeling by An Ly.
Bottom: Hairstyling and photography by Christina Butcher, modeling by Nicole Jeyaraj.

HOW TO GET IT

WHAT YOU NEED

- Brush
- Hair clip
- Hair elastic
- Bobby pins
- Hairspray (optional)

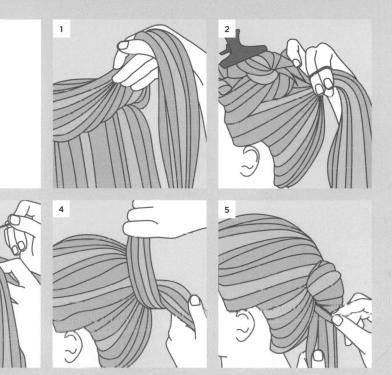

1. Brush your hair to remove any knots. Take a section of hair at the top of your head to your crown and clip it up and out of the way.

2. Gather the remainder of your hair into a ponytail at your crown. Try to place the base of the ponytail close to the edge of the section you clipped up at the top. Secure your ponytail with a hair elastic.

3. Next, unclip the top section of hair and adjust the front to sit in a small pompadour shape. Use a bobby pin to secure in place just above your ponytail.

4. Wrap the remainder of the top section of hair around your ponytail. Stay as close to the base of your ponytail as possible to avoid the hair sliding down as you wrap it around. Secure the end of the wrapped section with a bobby pin.

5. Flatten your ponytail against the back of your head and use bobby pins to secure it in place.

TOP TIP

To get a neat, smooth finish, hold the end of your ponytail while you adjust the wrapped section so that it sits flat against the back of your head. Angle your bobby pins diagonally, and for a stronger hold you can cross your pins in an X shape. Finish with hairspray to keep your ponytail in place.

FLIPPED-OVER PONYTAIL
THE LOOK

Turn the classic ponytail on its head with this flipped-over ponytail. By turning the base of the ponytail inside out and pushing it through itself, you can add body to your ponytail and give it a new dimension. The knot or bun that you're left with at the base of the ponytail is its own accessory, though a flower corsage or ribbon can be added for a touch of color. Perfect for school, work, or going out with friends, this style is a pretty alternative to a regular ponytail.

DIFFICULTY LEVEL
Easy

IDEAL HAIR LENGTH
Medium to long

HAIR EXTENSIONS NEEDED?
No

ASSISTANCE NEEDED?
No

ACCESSORIES
Use hair elastics that match the color of your hair to keep them inconspicuous. Add a pin or flower corsage in between the flip for an elegant or formal look.

TRY THIS
Combine this technique with the bobble ponytail (see pages 20–21) for an almost-braided ponytail look.

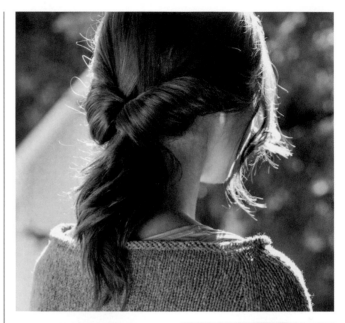

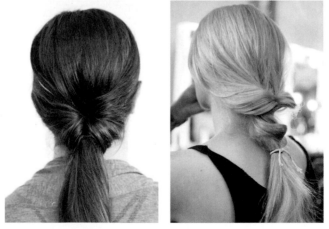

 SEE ALSO
Quiffed ponytail, pages 08–09
Bobble ponytail, pages 20–21

Top: Photograph courtesy of Brooklyn Tweed. Hairstyling by Véronik Avery, photography by Jared Flood, modeling by Stephanie Gelot.
Bottom left: Hairstyling and photography by Marie-Pierre Sander.
Bottom right: Hairstyling and photography by Christina Butcher, modeling by Fiana Stewart.

HOW TO GET IT

WHAT YOU NEED

- Brush
- Hair elastic
- Topsy Tail tool

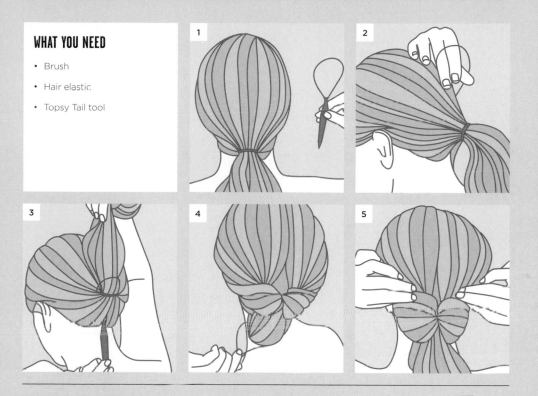

1. Brush your hair to remove any knots. Gather your hair into a ponytail at the back of your head or sitting low above your neck and secure it with an elastic.

2. Take your Topsy Tail tool and place it in your hair above your ponytail elastic.

3. Pull your ponytail up through the loop of the Topsy Tail tool.

4. While holding the end of your ponytail up, pull the Topsy Tail down. You may need to adjust it as your hair elastic is flipped over. Keep pulling your hair down until it is all the way through.

5. Adjust the twisted sections to sit neatly.

TOP TIP

It's possible to do this style without the Topsy Tail: simply use your fingers to make a space above your hair elastic and flip your ponytail through. Alternatively, you can DIY your own tool with fabric-covered wire.

STACKED PONYTAIL
THE LOOK

This sleek, sectioned ponytail is an elegant take on the classic low ponytail. Recently seen on Fashion Week catwalks, this style can take your everyday ponytail from ordinary to extraordinary. Good for both daytime and nighttime wear, this pony style maintains your hair length while at the same time giving it a stylishly simple look.

DIFFICULTY LEVEL
Easy

IDEAL HAIR LENGTH
Long

HAIR EXTENSIONS NEEDED?
No, but you can use a ponytail extension to add length.

ASSISTANCE NEEDED?
No

ACCESSORIES
Use clear elastics or try colored hair ties for a fun variation. For nighttime you could add a jeweled ponytail clip at the base.

TRY THIS
You can create a stack of four or five ponytails by taking smaller sections down the back of your head. You could even continue down your ponytail the same as in the bobble ponytail (see pages 20-21).

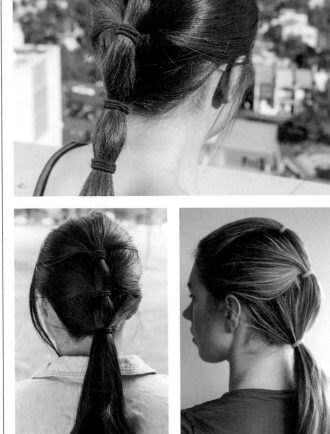

▶ **SEE ALSO**
Bobble ponytail, pages 20–21
Coiled bun, pages 76-77

Top: Hairstyling and photography by Christina Butcher, modeling by Adeline Er.
Bottom left: Hairstyling and photography by Christina Butcher, modeling by Willa Zheng.
Bottom right: Hairstyling, photography, and modeling by Christina Butcher.

HOW TO GET IT

WHAT YOU NEED

- Brush
- 3 hair elastics
- Hair serum
- Hairspray

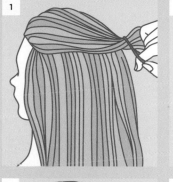

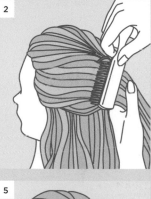

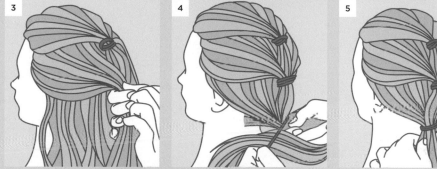

1. Make a ponytail at the top of your head with a one-third section of hair, and secure with an elastic.

2. Brush back the next section of hair at ear level to create a ponytail at the back of your head, incorporating the first ponytail.

3. Secure this second section with a hair elastic.

4. Gather all your hair into a ponytail at the nape of your neck and secure with an elastic.

5. Smooth your ponytail with serum and finish with a light mist of hairspray to catch any flyaways

TOP TIP

Spray hairspray onto your brush, rather than your hair, then lightly brush to catch those fine flyaway hairs. If you have layers, curl the ends of your hair under so that they don't stick out of your ponytail.

TWIST-OVER PONYTAIL
THE LOOK

Put beautiful detail into your hair with this style. Creating small rope twists that join into the main ponytail adds a cosmopolitan, chic look to the regular ponytail. This look is perfect for the social scene —just get ready for everyone asking how you did it! This twist-over ponytail works if you have layers in your hair, as long as they reach your ponytail. Try a ponytail extension to give you a fuller look.

DIFFICULTY LEVEL
Medium

IDEAL HAIR LENGTH
Medium to long

HAIR EXTENSIONS NEEDED?
No, but you can use a ponytail extension on shorter hair.

ASSISTANCE NEEDED?
No

ACCESSORIES
You don't really need to add accessories to this look, as there is enough pretty detail in the twisted sections. This low hairstyle is perfect under a hat or headband.

TRY THIS
Instead of twisting each section, try simple braids. They will add more texture to the style. Alternatively, split the side sections into more subsections—try four or even five small twisted sections to add into the ponytail to create a more intricate look.

▶ **SEE ALSO**
Flipped-over ponytail, pages 12–13
Figure-8 braid, pages 44–45

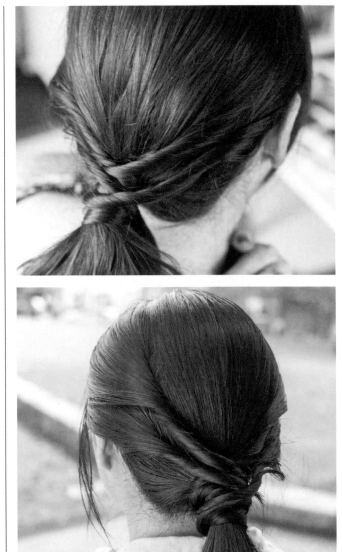

Top: Hairstyling and photography by Christina Butcher, modeling by Monica Richmond.
Bottom: Hairstyling and photography by Christina Butcher, modeling by Willa Zheng.

HOW TO GET IT

WHAT YOU NEED

- Brush
- Hair clips
- Hair elastic
- Bobby pins

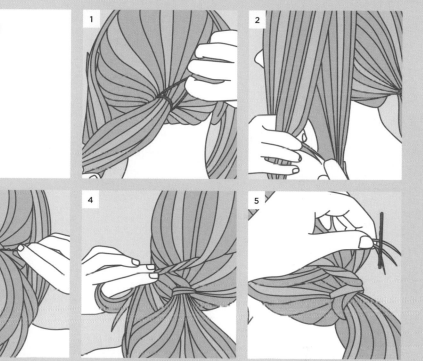

1. Brush your hair through to remove any knots or tangles. Clip away two medium-sized sections of hair, one on either side of your face. Put the rest of your hair in a ponytail and secure with a hair elastic.

2. Separate each side section into three equal parts.

3. Starting with the lowest section, twist the hair into a rope and then wrap it around your ponytail. Secure the end with a bobby pin.

4. Repeat on the other side, then go on to the middle section, and so on.

5. Continue twisting each section and pin in place around your ponytail with bobby pins until you're done.

TOP TIP

A trick for keeping your hair in place is to tease the end of each section, wrap it around the elastic, and then pin in place. Putting the pin on the end of your hair first will make this much easier. Curling your hair before wrapping it around the ponytail will stop your ends sticking out.

1960s PONYTAIL
THE LOOK

Channel your inner Bardot with this retro-inspired ponytail. The crown is lightly teased to create volume and the ponytail sits low at the back of the head. The curved ends to the ponytail give this style that '60s glam look.

DIFFICULTY LEVEL
Easy

IDEAL HAIR LENGTH
Long

HAIR EXTENSIONS NEEDED?
No, but you can use a ponytail extension on medium-length hair.

ASSISTANCE NEEDED?
No

ACCESSORIES
If you have bangs you can use a pretty pin to clip them back. Sideswept bangs will embrace that '60s feel.

TRY THIS
Keep it loose and messy for a Brigitte Bardot feel, and wear with winged eyeliner. For a chic, evening updo, twist the ponytail into a chignon at the nape of your neck.

▶ **SEE ALSO**
Quiffed ponytail, pages 08–09
Classic 1960s bouffant, pages 86–87

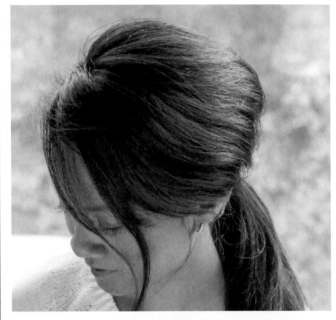

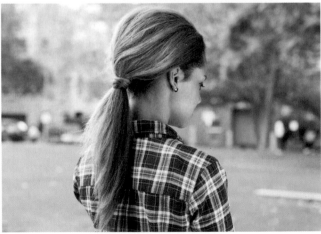

Top: Hairstyling and photography by Christina Butcher, modeling by Patricia Almario. Bottom: Hairstyling by Christina Butcher, photography by Xiaohan Shen, modeling by Dorothy Jean Joly.

HOW TO GET IT

WHAT YOU NEED

- Bristle brush or comb
- Hairspray (optional)
- Hair elastic
- Bobby pins

1. Separate your hair into top and bottom sections. Create volume and a bouffant shape with the top section by teasing at the crown of your head using a comb or bristle brush. Add a little hairspray if you need extra hold.

2. Gather all your hair into a low ponytail and secure with a hair elastic. Don't pull the hair too tightly, as you want to keep as much volume as possible in the crown area. Gently pull at the top of your ponytail to loosen the hair and create a 1960s silhouette.

3. Using the bristle brush or comb, smooth over the top section of hair to create a rounder shape.

4. Take a small piece of hair from the base of your ponytail and wrap it around your hair elastic to cover it.

5. Secure the ends of the wrapped hair underneath with a bobby pin.

TOP TIP

It's important to start this style with a strong base and, depending on your hair type, you will need some product to create volume. Try a volumizer or mousse in towel-dried hair and blow-dry with a round brush. If your hair is wavy, second-day hair will hold this style well.

BOBBLE PONYTAIL
THE LOOK

With such a distinctive shape, the sectioned bobble ponytail is fun but sleek and is so easy to do. Puff out each section of the ponytail to give it a unique look. This style combines the functionality of keeping your hair well and truly under control with a cute look that's perfect for a day out with friends.

DIFFICULTY LEVEL
Easy

IDEAL HAIR LENGTH
Long

HAIR EXTENSIONS NEEDED?
No, but you can use a ponytail extension on shorter hair.

ASSISTANCE NEEDED?
No

ACCESSORIES
For a more streamlined look, use hair elastics that match your hair color. Alternatively, why not try metallic hair elastics or hair cuffs as a feature, or use colored hair ties for a fun finish.

TRY THIS
This hairstyle is particularly effective in straight hair, but it can also be worn in wavy or curly hair. Why not combine the bobble ponytail with the stacked ponytail (see pages 14–15)? Section your hair down the back of your head and continue into a low bobble ponytail at the nape of your neck. You can also wear this hairstyle to the side or twist it into a top knot bun.

▶ **SEE ALSO**
Rope twist, pages 54–55
Top knot bun, pages 64–65

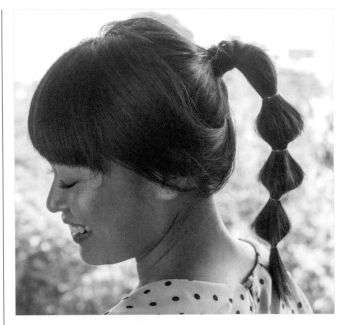

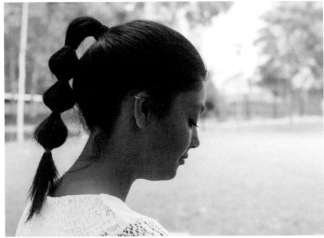

Top: Hairstyling and photography by Christina Butcher, modeling by Carolyn Mach.
Bottom: Hairstyling and photography by Christina Butcher, modeling by Nicole Jeyaraj.

HOW TO GET IT

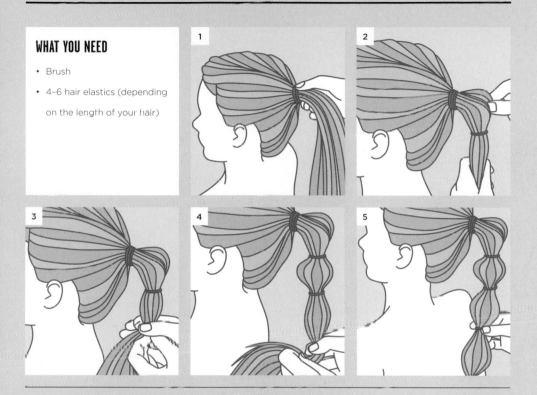

WHAT YOU NEED

- Brush
- 4–6 hair elastics (depending on the length of your hair)

1. Brush your hair to remove any knots. Gather all your hair into a ponytail at the back of your head and secure with an elastic. You can place the ponytail higher on the crown of your head if you're after a bouncier look.

2. Next, take a hair elastic and place it around your ponytail about 2 inches from the base of your ponytail.

3. Continue placing hair elastics in equal measures down the length of your ponytail.

4. Keep going!

5. When you're done, gently pull at each section of hair to stretch it out and emphasize the shape.

TOP TIP

Gently pulling at each section of hair not only emphasizes the distinctive shape of this ponytail, but also makes your hair look thicker.

BASIC BRAID
THE LOOK

The basic braid is also known as a plait. It is the main building block you'll use for all braiding styles, but it's also a beautiful hairstyle on its own. It involves weaving three sections of hair together and repeating this process to form the braid. This is one of the most versatile techniques and looks great in all hair types. This chapter will show you examples of how this technique can be used to create a number of different looks.

DIFFICULTY LEVEL
Easy

IDEAL HAIR LENGTH
Medium to long

HAIR EXTENSIONS NEEDED?
No

ASSISTANCE NEEDED?
No

ACCESSORIES
Team the braid with a ribbon for a cute finish, or use flowers for a bohemian look.

TRY THIS
You can wear the basic braid anywhere in your hair. Wear it to the back or over your shoulder to the side.

▶ **SEE ALSO**
Braided headband, pages 28–29
Heidi braids, pages 42–43

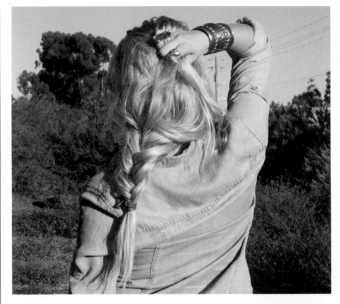

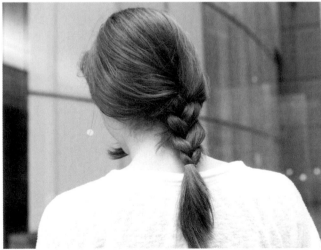

Top: Hairstyling, photography, and modeling by Emily Goswick.
Bottom: Hairstyling by Christina Butcher, photography by Xiaohan Shen, modeling by Laura Muheim.

HOW TO GET IT

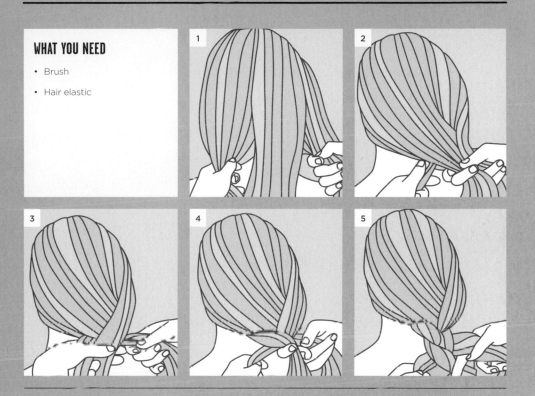

WHAT YOU NEED

- Brush
- Hair elastic

1. Brush your hair to remove any knots and split your hair into three equal pieces.

2. Take the piece on the left and cross it over the middle. Next, take the piece on the right and cross it over the left (now middle) piece. You'll start to see the braid forming.

3. Take the section now on the left and cross it over the middle and then repeat again, bringing the right over the left (now middle).

4. As you continue down, bring each outer piece over the middle to keep forming the braid.

5. When you're finished, secure the end of your hair with an elastic.

TOP TIP

Using small clear elastics will help when creating braided hairstyles, as the band won't show through the finished upstyle. Pull gently at the sides of your braid to loosen it and stretch it out. This will make your hair look thicker and emphasize the shape.

FRENCH BRAID
THE LOOK

The French braid is a classic, timeless hairstyle. It is created by initially following the basic braid technique and then adding in small sections of hair from each side as you continue down the back of your head. The French braid sits close to your head and is a beautiful way to wear your hair up. It looks great in curly, wavy, and straight hair types and suits all hair lengths, from shoulder length to extremely long hair.

DIFFICULTY LEVEL
Medium

IDEAL HAIR LENGTH
Medium to long

HAIR EXTENSIONS NEEDED?
No

ASSISTANCE NEEDED?
Yes, but you can do this in your own hair with practice.

ACCESSORIES
Thread ribbon through as you braid to accentuate the structure or use a decorative hair elastic at the end of the braid for a pretty finish.

TRY THIS
Once you've mastered the French braid style, you can move it around to create an infinite number of hairstyles. Try a half braid, diagonal braid, S-shaped braid, or an upside-down braid bun.

▶ **SEE ALSO**
Waterfall braid, pages 58–59
Upside-down braid bun, pages 74–75

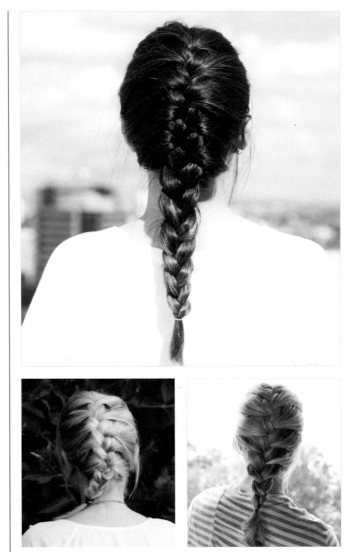

Top: Hairstyling by Christina Butcher, photography by Xiaohan Shen, modeling by Sophia Phan.
Bottom left: Hairstyling, photography, and modeling by Suzy Wimbourne Photography.
Bottom right: Hairstyling and modeling by Christina Butcher, photography by Xiaohan Shen.

HOW TO GET IT

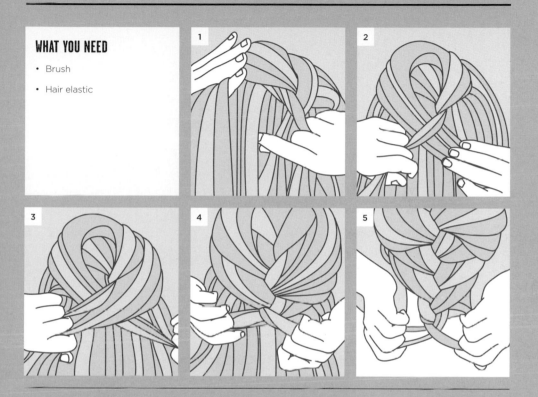

WHAT YOU NEED

- Brush
- Hair elastic

1. Start by taking a section of hair at the top of your head and splitting it into three equal pieces. In the same way that you form a regular braid, bring the left section over the middle and the right over the left (now middle).

2. When you bring your left over the middle again, grab a little extra piece of hair from the left side of your head, combine it with the left section, and bring them into the middle together.

3. Then, on the right side, bring that section over the middle and add in another piece of hair from the right-hand side. This way you keep forming a regular braid but you add in sections of hair as you go.

4. Continue down the back of your head, adding in equal sections of hair to your braid.

5. Once all your hair is added, finish in a basic braid and secure the end with a hair elastic.

TOP TIP

To keep your braid straight, be aware of your dominant hand—if you're right-handed, concentrate on your left hand. Also, look down as you braid. If your head is turned, the braid won't be straight. Make sure you keep the sections that you add in even, and keep the braid taut as you work.

DUTCH BRAID
THE LOOK

Now that you've practiced creating both a basic braid and a French braid, you can move on to the Dutch braid! This style is just the reverse of a French braid, and is sometimes called an inside-out braid. Instead of bringing pieces over and into the middle, you bring them under and into the middle so that the braid sits on top. This style suits straight hair, but also looks great in curly hair.

DIFFICULTY LEVEL
Medium

IDEAL HAIR LENGTH
Medium to long

HAIR EXTENSIONS NEEDED?
No

ASSISTANCE NEEDED?
Yes, but you can do this in your own hair with practice.

ACCESSORIES
Like with the French braid, you can add ribbons or bows for a sweet look, or add flowers for a bohemian twist.

TRY THIS
This versatile technique can be used in many hairstyles and can be varied to create an infinite number of looks. Try braiding your hair diagonally downward or into an upside-down braid bun (see pages 74–75).

▶ **SEE ALSO**
Cornrows, pages 50–51
Lace braid, pages 60–61

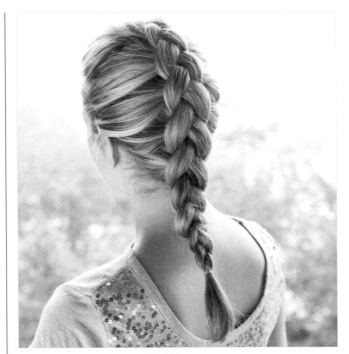

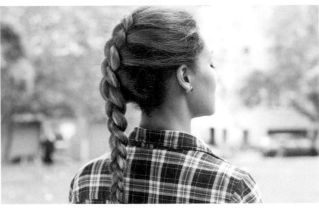

Top: Hairstyling, photography, and modeling by Christina Butcher.
Bottom: Hairstyling by Christina Butcher, photography by Xiaohan Shen, modeling by Dorothy Jean Joly.

HOW TO GET IT

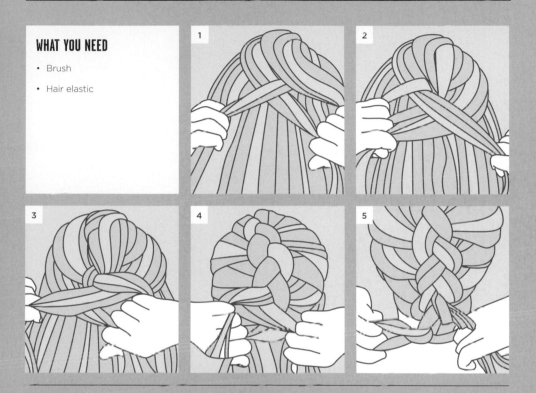

WHAT YOU NEED

- Brush
- Hair elastic

1. Take a section of hair at the top of your head and split it into three equal pieces. Begin braiding by taking the left piece under the middle piece and the right piece under the left (now middle) piece.

2. Bring the left piece under the middle again, and add in a small section of hair from the left side.

3. Continue on the right, bringing the right piece under, and adding in a small section of hair from the right-hand side. This way you'll keep forming a reverse braid, but adding in sections of hair underneath as you go.

4. Continue down the back of your head, adding in equal sections of hair to your braid.

5. Once all your hair is added, finish in a reverse braid and secure the end with a hair elastic.

TOP TIP

This braid takes some practice, but you'll find it will hold in your hair longer than a French braid because the layers don't need to reach over the top. The Dutch braid looks best when it has been stretched out. It has a nicer shape and will give the impression of thicker hair.

BRAIDED HEADBAND
THE LOOK

Create the perfect hair accessory using your own hair! Two hidden braids taken from behind your ears cross over the top of your head to form a braided headband. This is a delicate-looking braid, but can be remarkably secure. It adds a countryside feel to your look and so is great for a picnic or spending the day outdoors with friends.

DIFFICULTY LEVEL
Medium

IDEAL HAIR LENGTH
Medium to long

HAIR EXTENSIONS NEEDED?
No

ASSISTANCE NEEDED?
No

ACCESSORIES
Your own hair is the accessory in this hairstyle, so no other adornment is needed. However, you could weave flowers or a ribbon through your headband to add an extra dimension to the finished look.

TRY THIS
If you have very long hair, you can just do one braid and cross it over the top of your head. If you have shorter hair, doing two braids makes the headband fuller and the style will look more even.

This style suits straight hair but looks great with wavy or curly hair too. You could also curl the rest of your hair and leave it out or tie it back into a loose bun.

▶ **SEE ALSO**
   Heidi braids, pages 42–43
   Lace braid, pages 60–61

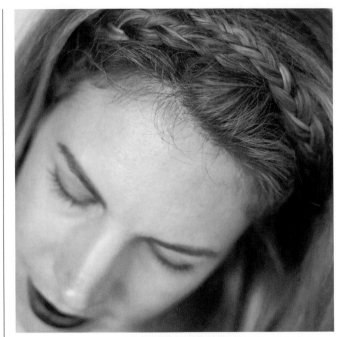

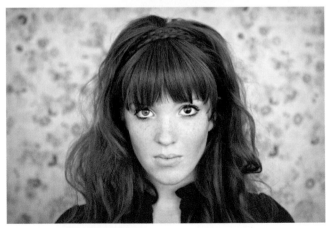

Top: Hairstyling, photography, and modeling by Christina Butcher.
Bottom: Hairstyling, photography, and modeling by Emily M. Meyers/The Freckled Fox.

HOW TO GET IT

WHAT YOU NEED

- Brush
- Hair clip
- 2 small clear hair elastics
- Bobby pins

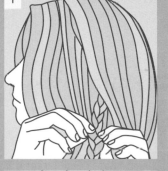

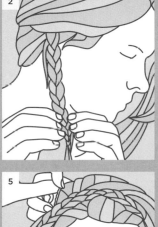

1. Start by brushing all your hair to remove any knots. Clip your hair back and take a 1-inch section of hair from behind your left ear. Braid this section and secure the end with a small clear elastic. Pull at the sides of the braid to loosen it and stretch it out. If you start pulling the braid just above the hair elastic and work back up, you can really enhance the shape of the braid and make your hair look thicker.

2. Repeat on your right side, braiding a 1-inch section of hair behind your right ear. Remember to stretch out your braid.

3-4. Pull one of the braids over your head and into a headband position, and pin in place on top of your hair.

5. Cross the other braid over and pin in place. Tuck the ends of both braids under each other and pin them down to hide them away, and then pin the two braids together for added hold.

TOP TIP

If you have long hair, you may only need to braid on one side of the head to achieve a full headband. Try to braid over the top of your head where the braids will eventually sit; if you start the braids in a downward direction, they won't sit as flat.

ANGEL BRAID
THE LOOK

The angel braid is made up of half a French braid, where you only add in hair from one side. Typically, this style is worn along your hairline to keep your hair away from your face. This pretty style can be adapted to sit along the side of your hair or farther back.

DIFFICULTY LEVEL
Medium

IDEAL HAIR LENGTH
Medium to long

HAIR EXTENSIONS NEEDED?
No

ASSISTANCE NEEDED?
No

ACCESSORIES
Your braid acts as a headband in this style, so there's no need for any additional accessories.

TRY THIS
This style looks great in both curly and straight hair. The braid doesn't have to sit at your hairline; try wearing it at the top of your head for a larger headband braid style, or curving it all around into a crowning braid (see pages 48–49).

▶ **SEE ALSO**
Braided headband, pages 28–29
Heart-shaped angel braid, pages 40–41

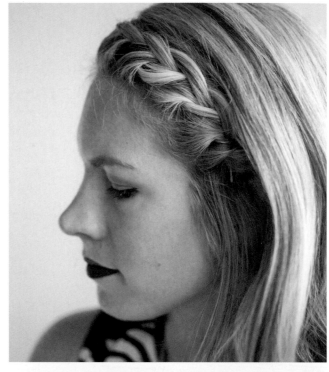

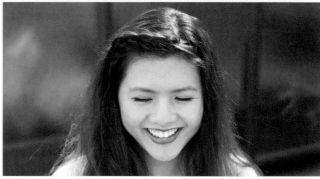

Top: Hairstyling, photography, and modeling by Christina Butcher.
Bottom: Hairstyling by Christina Butcher, photography by Xiaohan Shen, modeling by Sophia Phan.

HOW TO GET IT

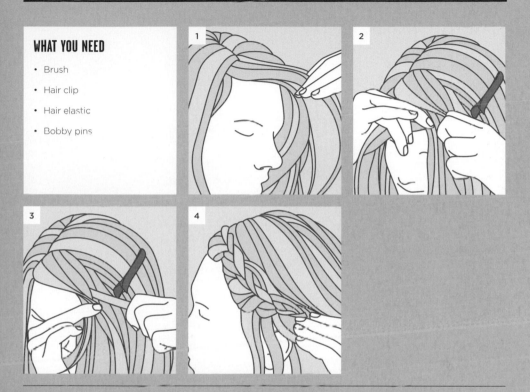

WHAT YOU NEED

- Brush
- Hair clip
- Hair elastic
- Bobby pins

1. Using a brush, make a deep side part on one side of your hair.

2. Section off a 1- to 2-inch section of hair along your hairline. Clip the rest of your hair back out of the way.

3. Split the section in three and start to French braid (see pages 24–25). Instead of adding hair in on both sides of the braid, however, just add in hair from the front. This will add height and create the braid along your hairline, and allow the rest of your hair to sit neatly behind it.

4. Continue to braid down to your ear, adding hair from the front, then finish in a basic braid and secure the end with a hair elastic. Angle the braid back behind your ear and pin in place with bobby pins. Arrange your hair over the top of the end of the braid to hide it.

TOP TIP

If you have bangs, you may end up with layers poking out of the braid. To disguise them, put a bobby pin on the ends of the hair that's sticking out and pin it behind and under the braid to hide them. If you have fine hair, you can lightly tease the top of your hair so the end of the braid is hidden.

FISHTAIL BRAID
THE LOOK

This braid is a favorite for long hair because it looks elaborate and difficult but is surprisingly easy to master. The fishtail braid is also referred to as the herringbone or fishbone braid, and is formed by sectioning your hair in two and then crossing over small sections of hair from side to side. It works beautifully in upstyles, as the unique texture adds a stunning twist to buns or chignons.

DIFFICULTY LEVEL
Medium

IDEAL HAIR LENGTH
Long

HAIR EXTENSIONS NEEDED?
No

ASSISTANCE NEEDED?
Yes

ACCESSORIES
The ultimate bohemian look is a messy fishtail braid and a flower crown—nothing too neat or precise with this loose hairstyle.

TRY THIS
Try twisting your fishtail braid into a chignon. The fishtail also adds a unique texture to buns and updos. Stretch the sides of your braid out to create a messy and bohemian look, or make three fishtails and braid them together.

▶ **SEE ALSO**
Fishtail braided bun, pages 66–67
Fishtail chignon, pages 82–83

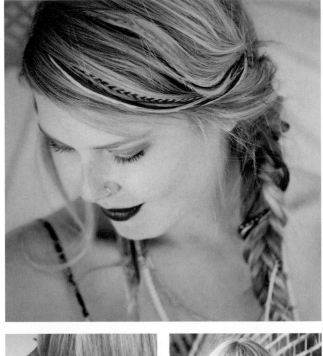

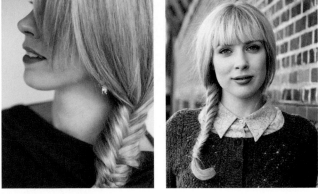

Top: Photograph courtesy of Fine Featherheads. Photography by Kate Broussard, Soulshots Photography.
Bottom left: Hairstyling, photography, and modeling by Christina Butcher.
Bottom right: Photograph courtesy of Brooklyn Tweed. Hairstyling by Karen Schaupeter, photography by Jared Flood, modeling by Hannah Metz.

HOW TO GET IT

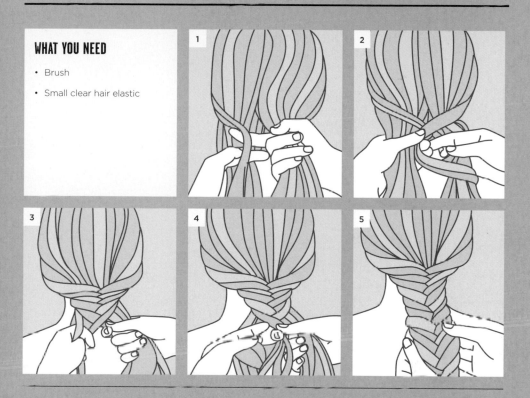

WHAT YOU NEED

- Brush
- Small clear hair elastic

1. Brush your hair to remove any knots. Split your hair into two equal sections. Hold one side in each hand and keep these separate as you braid.

2. Take a small piece of hair from the left side of the left ponytail and cross it over to the right ponytail.

3. Repeat on the right. Take a small piece of hair from the right side of the right ponytail and cross it over to the left ponytail.

4. Repeat this process all the way down your hair. Each time, cross a small piece of hair from one side to the other. As you move down your hair, the pieces will cross over to form the fishtail braid.

5. Secure the end of your fishtail braid with a small clear elastic. Gently pull at the sides of the braid to stretch it out. This will make your hair look thicker and fuller, and emphasize the shape of the braid.

TOP TIP

When you're learning to fishtail braid, it's easier to put your hair up in a ponytail. This is also helpful for keeping your braid in place, especially if you have layers. Doing the fishtail braid while your hair is wet will also make it easier to hold and allow you to be more precise.

BOW BRAIDS
THE LOOK

Wow your friends with these stunning bow braids. You can integrate the bow braid into almost any style with a French or lace braid technique. This braid is suitable for all hair lengths and layered hair, but works best in straight hair. Make sure to have your answers at the ready though, because everyone will be asking how you did your hair!

DIFFICULTY LEVEL
Hard

IDEAL HAIR LENGTH
Medium to long

HAIR EXTENSIONS NEEDED?
No

ASSISTANCE NEEDED?
Yes

ACCESSORIES
Your hair provides the bows for this style, so there's no need to add any further adornments.

TRY THIS
There are so many ways to use this bow technique in braids and upstyles. Wherever you can do a French braid, you can transform it into bow braids. Simply leave a slim section of hair loose along the edge of your French braid to form the bows. You can try a bow-braided headband, diagonal braid, or bow-braided pigtails.

▶ **SEE ALSO**
Pretzel braid, pages 62–63
Bow bun, pages 78–79

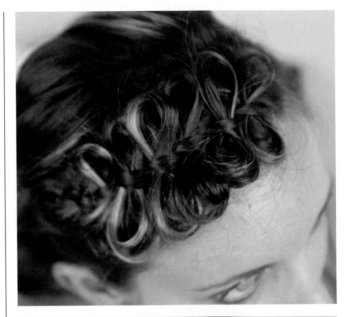

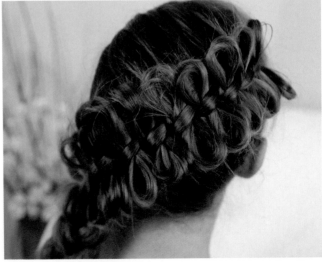

Top and bottom: Hairstyling, photography, and modeling by Mindy McKnight.

HOW TO GET IT

WHAT YOU NEED

- Brush
- Fine comb
- Hairspray or pomade
- Hairpin
- Hair elastics

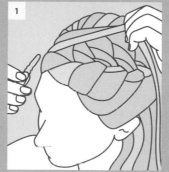

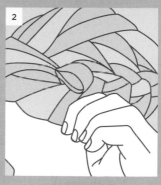

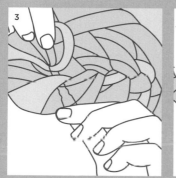

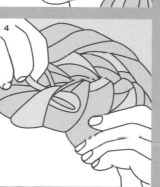

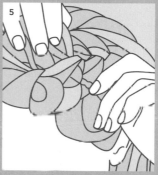

1. Begin by braiding a section of your hair. You can use an angel braid (see pages 30–31) or a French braid (see pages 24–25). Leave a ½-inch section of hair loose, adjacent to your braid, to create the bow.

2. Take a small piece of hair from the ½-inch section and circle it around your finger to create a loop. Place your hairpin, closed end first, through a section of your braid.

3. Thread the loop of hair through the end of your hairpin and take the loop of hair with your left hand while gently pulling the hairpin back through your braid with your right hand.

4. As you bring the hairpin back out of your braid, it will create the other half of the bow. Gently pull the hairpin until you like the look of the second loop and then remove it from your hair. You should now have one completed bow that runs through the braid.

5. Repeat steps 2 to 4 until you run out of hair.

TOP TIP

Depending on the length of your hair, you may have some leftover hair trailing out after making each bow. You can either combine this tail section of hair with the next piece or leave it laying alongside the braid. The next bow loop will cover the loose pieces, so they won't be so obvious.

BRAIDED KNOT BUNS
THE LOOK

A braided variation on the classic French twist (see pages 70-71), this row of mini braided buns creates a knotted effect down the back of your head. This style looks complicated, but it's not that difficult to do. Working in small, separate sections is key to managing this intriguing style. This updo is made up of four stacked ponytails, one on top of the other at the back of your head, and each bun is independent. You only need to know how to do a basic braid (see pages 22-23) to create this hairstyle. Similar to mini buns (see pages 84-85), this style is more suited to long or thicker hair.

DIFFICULTY LEVEL
Medium

IDEAL HAIR LENGTH
Medium to long

HAIR EXTENSIONS NEEDED?
No

ASSISTANCE NEEDED?
No

ACCESSORIES
The detail in the braided knot buns means that you don't need to add any hair accessories in this style. If you have bangs or layers, use a jeweled clip to pin them back, away from your face.

TRY THIS
If your hair is fine or short, try mini buns instead. Alternatively, customize the style to suit your hair.

▶ **SEE ALSO**
  Bow bun, pages 78-79
  Mini buns, pages 84-85

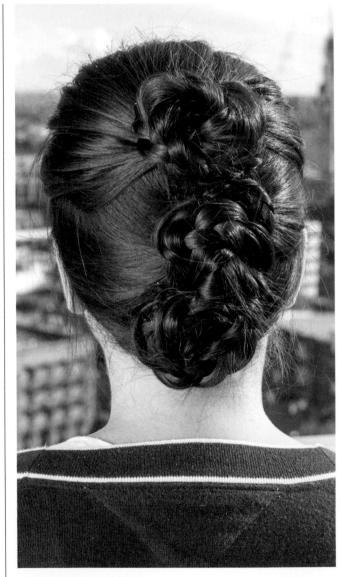

Hairstyling and photography by Christina Butcher, modeling by An Ly.

HOW TO GET IT

WHAT YOU NEED

- Brush
- 8 small clear hair elastics
  (2 per braided bun)
- Bobby pins

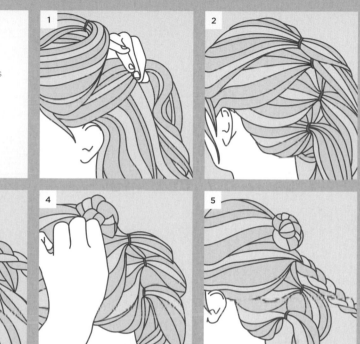

1. Start by brushing all your hair back. You can leave your bangs loose or include them in the style. Take a section of hair running from about your temple back and secure it with a hair elastic.

2. Next, take a section between your temple and your ear and pull it back to make another ponytail section. Secure with a hair elastic. Pull back a third section of hair just level with the back of your ears and make a third ponytail. Gather the rest of your hair into a ponytail directly underneath the other sections you have just made. You should have four ponytails.

3. Braid the top ponytail and secure the end of your braid with an elastic.

4. Wrap the braid around itself and pin in place to make a little bun.

5. Repeat this with the three remaining ponytails to form a vertical row of braided buns.

TOP TIP

Using clear elastics for this style is best, as they don't protrude from the buns and will create a seamless finish. With so many sections, each braid can look a bit thin on its own, so make sure to stretch them out to make them look thicker.

SCARF PIGTAILS
THE LOOK

In this style a scarf becomes a special feature. It sits like a headband across the top of your head and is then used as a section in each pigtail braid, helping to make your hair look thicker. The scarf can be used to add color to your hair, or to complement whatever you're wearing. Straight or curly hair looks great in this style.

DIFFICULTY LEVEL
Medium

IDEAL HAIR LENGTH
Medium to long

HAIR EXTENSIONS NEEDED?
No

ASSISTANCE NEEDED?
No

ACCESSORIES
Large rectangular scarfs are easy to work into this style, but if you have a square scarf, simply fold it diagonally until you get a 2-inch-wide strip. The style of your scarf will transform the look of this braid. Pick a neutral tone for an elegant style or a bright, colorful scarf for a fun look.

TRY THIS
Pigtails not your thing? This style looks gorgeous with the braids pinned up at the nape of your neck. Fold the braid up, tucking the ends under, and pin in place. Pin the second braid over the top of the first for a beautiful braided updo.

▶ **SEE ALSO**
Dutch braid, pages 26–27
Waterfall braid, pages 58–59

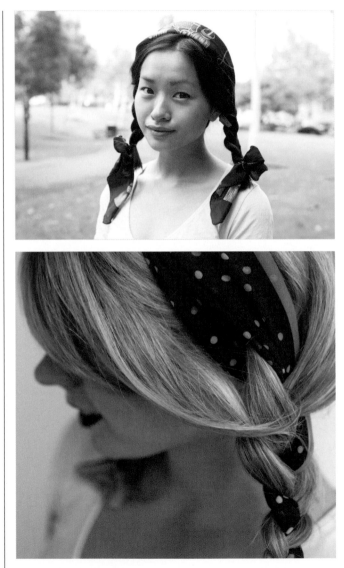

Top: Hairstyling by Christina Butcher, photography by Xiaohan Shen, modeling by Jessica Tran.
Bottom: Hairstyling, photography, and modeling by Christina Butcher.

HOW TO GET IT

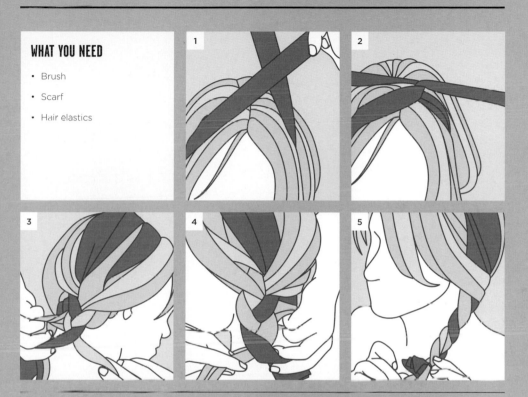

WHAT YOU NEED

- Brush
- Scarf
- Hair elastics

1. Brush and loosely part your hair. Place the scarf around the back of your neck, and bring it up like a headband.

2. Twist the ends of the scarf around each other to form a turban-style knot.

3. Bring the ends of your scarf down on either side and make sure they're about the same length as your hair. Secure one side of your hair and one end of the scarf with a hair elastic (this helps keep the tension in the scarf and stops the knot from moving as you braid the other side).

4. The scarf will form one of the three sections of the regular braid. Split the rest of your hair in two and use the scarf as the center section, then just weave the two hair sections and the scarf into a regular braid and secure with a clear elastic.

5. Repeat on the other side.

TOP TIP

If your hair is very long, you may not need to put the scarf around the back of your head to do the first headband piece. Instead, you could place the scarf over your head, trailing the ends down on either side as part of the pigtails. You want the ends of the scarf to be level with your ends.

HEART-SHAPED ANGEL BRAID
THE LOOK

Love is in the hair! You can wear your heart in your hair with this romantic braided hairstyle. This look uses a technique similar to the angel braid to create a heart-shaped outline. Although it might seem impossible, this style isn't as hard to master as you'd think!

DIFFICULTY LEVEL
Medium

IDEAL HAIR LENGTH
Medium to long

HAIR EXTENSIONS NEEDED?
No

ASSISTANCE NEEDED?
Yes, but you can do this in your own hair with practice.

ACCESSORIES
Add a red or pink ribbon at the bottom of the heart for an extra-sweet finish.

TRY THIS
This heart stands out clearly on straight hair, but you can also curl the ends of your hair for a more romantic hairstyle. Instead of finishing in a half-up style, incorporate your heart-shaped angel braid into a low ponytail.

▶ **SEE ALSO**
Half-up heart braid, pages 56–57
Bow bun, pages 78–79

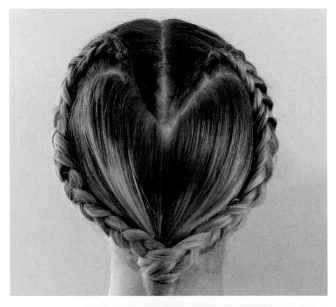

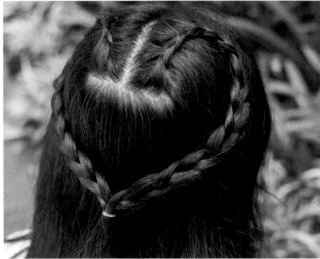

Top: Hairstyling, photography, and modeling by Jemma Grace.
Bottom: Hairstyling and photography by Christina Butcher, modeling by Riko Ishihata.

HOW TO GET IT

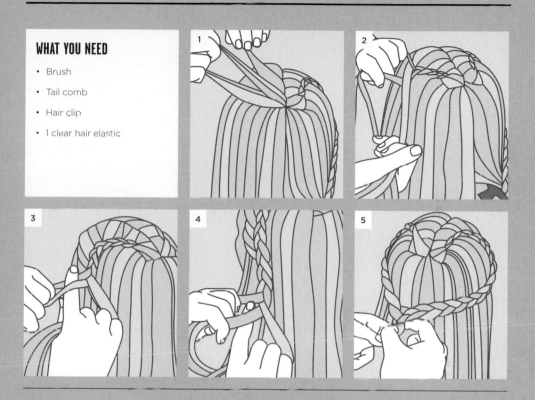

WHAT YOU NEED

- Brush
- Tail comb
- Hair clip
- 1 clear hair elastic

1. Brush your hair and create a deep center part with your tail comb. Use your hair clip to keep half your hair away while you do the first braid.

2. Make a horizontal part at the crown, running from your center part to your ear. Pick up a section of hair at the crown and split into three.

3. Begin your angel braid (see pages 30–31), angling it toward your face, only adding in hair on the outer side of the braid. After you have added about three pieces to the braid, turn the braid by angling it toward your ear to create the rounded top of the heart.

4. Continue braiding the heart shape, only adding in hair from the front until you reach the ear. At this point, stop adding hair and continue with a basic braid until you reach the middle of your head at your neckline. Secure with a hair elastic. Release the clip from the other side and repeat the angel braid on the other side to match the first.

5. Connect the two braids at the back of your head.

TOP TIP

To keep the heart shape even, only add in small sections to your braid. Keep the braids quite tight so that you can see where they're going and make adjustments as you go.

HEIDI BRAIDS
THE LOOK

Leave Heidi behind frolicking in the Swiss Alpine meadows! The sweet, girlish charm of this braided style is easily updated to a modern, wearable look. Best in long hair, Heidi braids are formed by making low pigtails and pinning the braids up and over to form a kind of headband. Pulling at the sides of the braids encourages your hair's natural texture and makes this hairstyle look modern.

DIFFICULTY LEVEL
Medium

IDEAL HAIR LENGTH
Long

HAIR EXTENSIONS NEEDED?
No

ASSISTANCE NEEDED?
No

ACCESSORIES
Heidi braids look beautiful accessorized with a scarf or ribbon. To do this, incorporate a scarf as one section of the braid and connect it across the back of your head to the other braid. You can also weave a ribbon through the finished style for added color.

TRY THIS
A center part is the classic look for this braid, but try varying the style with a side part or zigzag part. Instead of a regular braid, try a fishtail braid to create an intricate, on-trend look.

▶ **SEE ALSO**
Braided headband, pages 28–29
Scarf pigtails, pages 38–39

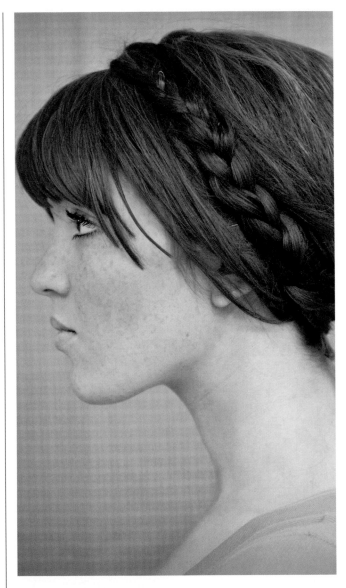

Hairstyling, photography, and modeling by Emily M. Meyers/The Freckled Fox.

HOW TO GET IT

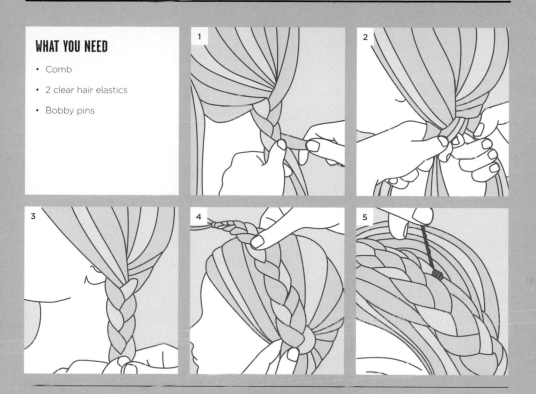

WHAT YOU NEED

- Comb
- 2 clear hair elastics
- Bobby pins

1. Using a comb, part your hair down the center from your forehead to the nape of your neck to create two equal sections.

2. Take the first section, split it into three equal sections, and make a basic braid, starting just behind your ear. Secure the end of your braid with a clear elastic.

3. Repeat, braiding the section on the other side.

4. Holding the start of your braid with one hand, pull the end of one braid up and over the top of your head. Pin in place with bobby pins.

5. Repeat with the second braid. Tuck the ends of both braids underneath each other, and secure with bobby pins. Place a couple of pins through both braids to join them together, and also pin the to the hair below so the style holds.

TOP TIP

When you are braiding, pull your hair down and slightly forward to keep it taut. This way, when you pull the braids up and over your head, you won't have too much loose hair at the back. Don't forget the braids are going up and over the top of your head, not down like most braids.

FIGURE-8 BRAID
THE LOOK

This intricate braid is also sometimes known as an infinity braid because the figure-8 pattern looks like the infinity symbol. To create this style, you'll horizontally wrap a small piece of hair in and around two sections of hair, forming the infinity "8" shape. In line with its design, the number of places you can wear this sleek, distinctive braid are limitless!

DIFFICULTY LEVEL
Medium

IDEAL HAIR LENGTH
Long

HAIR EXTENSIONS NEEDED?
No

ASSISTANCE NEEDED?
Yes

ACCESSORIES
To add some color, try tying a ribbon around one of the winding sections and weaving it through the braid. A simple bow or clip at the end of the braid is also a nice touch.

TRY THIS
This unique braid can be worn in a half-up style or as a side braid, and you can incorporate this braid in your hair wherever you would wear a fishtail braid. It also creates beautiful texture when twisted up into a bun.

▶ **SEE ALSO**
Fishtail braid, pages 32–33
Fishtail braided bun, pages 66–67

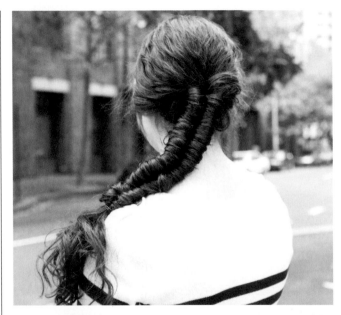

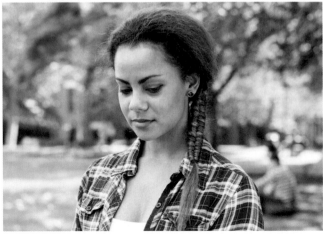

Top: Hairstyling by Christina Butcher, photography by Xiaohan Shen, modeling by Monica Bowerman .
Bottom: Hairstyling by Christina Butcher, photography by Xiaohan Shen, modeling by Dorothy Jean Joly.

HOW TO GET IT

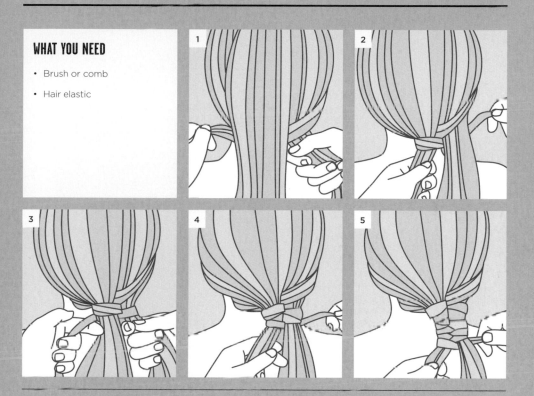

WHAT YOU NEED

- Brush or comb
- Hair elastic

1. Brush your hair to remove any knots. Split your hair into two equal sections. Take a small piece of hair from the outside of the right section and bring it over the right section and under the left section.

2. Next, bring the piece of hair over the left section and under the right section.

3. Continue in a figure-8 pattern, wrapping the piece of hair around the two sections.

4. When you start to run out of hair, add in another small piece of hair from the side and continue in the figure-8 shape.

5. Continue all the way down your hair and secure the end with an elastic.

TOP TIP

It's important to keep the looping figure-8 pattern tight as you braid. Keep the tension in the weaving piece of hair—this will keep the shape of the braid consistent.

GRECIAN BRAID
THE LOOK

Inspired by classics from the silver screen, this beautiful braid pays tribute to the elegance and simplicity of the ancient Greeks. You'll form this hairstyle by French braiding in a ring around the hairline, beginning at your right ear and braiding over your forehead, following your hairline until you run out of hair. Wear this braid in the sunshine—it's perfect for picnics, the beach, festivals . . . and toga parties!

DIFFICULTY LEVEL
Hard

IDEAL HAIR LENGTH
Medium to long

HAIR EXTENSIONS NEEDED?
No

ASSISTANCE NEEDED?
Yes, but you can do this in your own hair with practice.

ACCESSORIES
This eye-catching braid doesn't need hair accessories, but you can focus on other items, such as earrings or a necklace, to complement your hair.

TRY THIS
If your hair is very long, you can complete this look by winding the braid into a bun and pinning it at the back of your head. If you have shorter hair, keep the braid nearer your crown and you should be able to go full circle with the hair you have. This should also help the braid stay secure.

▶ **SEE ALSO**
French braid, pages 24–25
Crowning braid, pages 48–49

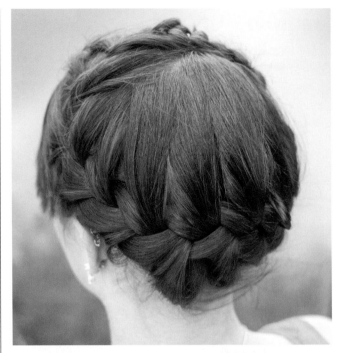

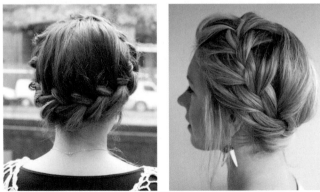

Top: Hairstyling and photography by Christina Butcher, modeling by Elly Hanson.
Bottom left: Hairstyling by Christina Butcher, photography by Xiaohan Shen, modeling by Teru Morihira.
Bottom right: Hairstyling, photography, and modeling by Christina Butcher.

HOW TO GET IT

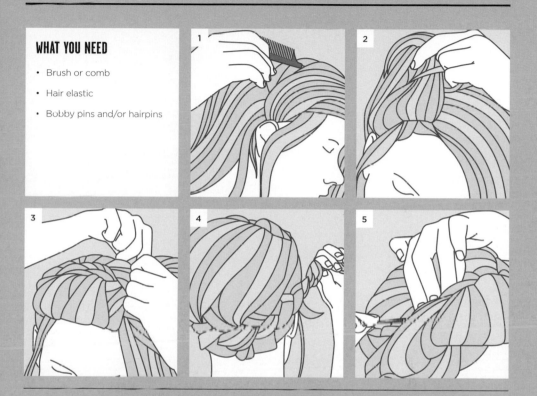

WHAT YOU NEED

- Brush or comb
- Hair elastic
- Bobby pins and/or hairpins

1. Take a section of hair above your right ear and split it into three.

2. Begin to French braid (see pages 24–25), adding in hair from both your hairline and from the crown behind. If you're left-handed, start at the top of your left ear and work round in the opposite direction to the instructions here. Using your stronger hand will help you make a neater braid.

3. Braid across your forehead and behind your left ear. As you reach the back of your left ear, keep following your hands around, keeping tension in the braid. Follow your hairline around the back of your head. By the time you reach the bottom right-hand side of your neck, you'll have added in all your hair.

4. Finish in a regular braid and secure with a small clear elastic.

5. Stretch out the braid, tuck the end under the start of the braid behind your right ear, and pin in place with bobby pins.

TOP TIP

If you like to have a little bit of height in the hair around your face, sit this braid about an inch back from your hairline. You can then gently stretch the braid out to adjust how your hair sits at the front. Use hairpins to pin the braid in place if you have long or thick hair.

CROWNING BRAID
THE LOOK

A pretty twist on a half-up hairstyle, crowning braids are formed by crossing over two braids at the back of your head. This style is an excellent look for weddings, whether you're part of the bridal party or a guest. Because all the detail is at the back, a veil or half veil looks beautiful pinned into the braids. This half-up, half-down style looks best with loose layers at the front and bangs left long and unstyled.

DIFFICULTY LEVEL
Medium

IDEAL HAIR LENGTH
Medium to long

HAIR EXTENSIONS NEEDED?
No

ASSISTANCE NEEDED?
No

ACCESSORIES
For a colorful twist, weave a fine ribbon through the finished braids so that it runs in and out of the inner edges. You can also use a headband or jeweled clip to pin back your bangs.

TRY THIS
Different techniques can add stunning detail to this simple style. Try other types of braids, such as the fishtail braid (see pages 32–33).

▶ **SEE ALSO**
Braided headband, pages 28–29
Half-up heart braid, pages 56–57

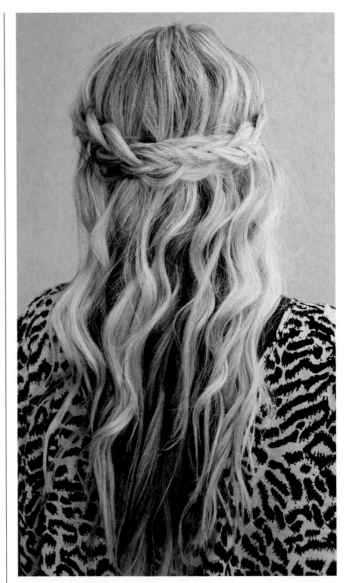

Hairstyling, photography, and modeling by Abby Smith/Twist Me Pretty.

HOW TO GET IT

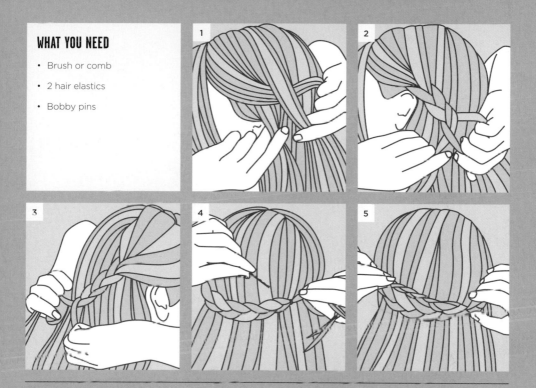

WHAT YOU NEED

- Brush or comb
- 2 hair elastics
- Bobby pins

1. Brush or comb your hair and part it down the middle. Gather two large sections of hair on each side of your face above your ears. Split one of the sections in three.

2. Begin braiding. Start loosely at the top, and angle your braid back. This way the braid will sit in the direction that you want the finished style to be. Secure the end of the braid with an elastic.

3. Repeat on the opposite side, making a braid above your other ear.

4. Cross the first braid behind your head and pin in place with bobby pins, making sure to tuck in the ends.

5. Cross the second braid behind your head and pin it level with the first braid, tucking the ends in underneath.

TOP TIP

If your braid is quite long, you can fold it in half and tuck the ends in behind the braid. To keep the two braids neat and close together as they cross, push pins in between the two braids so that they are connected and fixed down more securely. Pull the sides of the braids out to give them shape.

CORNROWS
THE LOOK

Cornrows are a traditional African hairstyle and braiding technique. These microbraids might be time-consuming, but they have a lot of impact and can last longer than other braided hairstyles. If you have the time, go for a full head of cornrows, or opt to integrate them into other hairstyles as an accent. Depending on how you wear them, cornrows look great for a big night out or a day in town with friends, and are especially great for the beach.

DIFFICULTY LEVEL
Medium to hard

IDEAL HAIR LENGTH
Any

HAIR EXTENSIONS NEEDED?
No

ASSISTANCE NEEDED?
Yes

ACCESSORIES
Cornrows are traditionally decorated with beads and shells.

TRY THIS
There are so many ways to incorporate cornrows into your favorite hairstyle. Try wearing them on the side to create a sweeping part, almost like an undercut. Depending on your skill level and patience, you can create patterns with your cornrows by zigzagging and deviating the braids as you go.

▶ **SEE ALSO**
Dutch braid, pages 26–27
Heart-shaped angel braid, pages 40–41

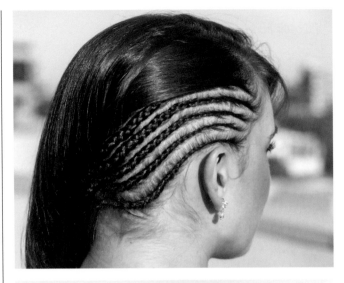

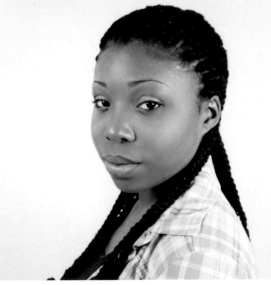

Top: Hairstyling and photography by Christina Butcher, modeling by Elly Hanson.
Bottom: Hairstyling, photography and modeling by Breanna Rutter/How To Black Hair LLC.

HOW TO GET IT

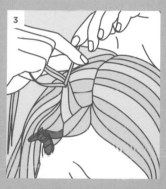

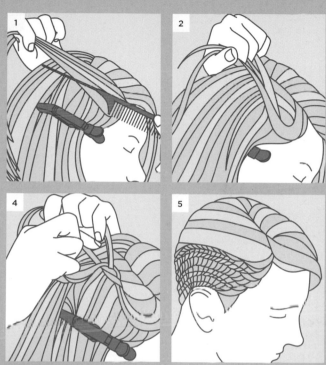

WHAT YOU NEED

- Tail comb
- Hair clips
- Small hair elastics
- Spray bottle filled with water (optional)

1. Use your tail comb to create a neat section for your cornrow braid. Clip the rest of your hair out of the way while you braid.

2. Split the start of the section in three and start to create a Dutch braid (see pages 26–27).

3. Add in small sections as you braid, always bringing the hair in from underneath.

4. When you have run out of hair, finish in a regular braid and secure the end with a small hair elastic.

5. Repeat over the rest of your head, making sure you take equal sections so that your cornrows are the same size.

TOP TIP

It takes time to get these braids to sit correctly. Practice with a larger braid and you will eventually master the technique. It helps to make neat sections, and to clip the rest of your hair away while you're working. Dampen your hair with water to make it more manageable.

FRENCH FISHTAIL BRAID
THE LOOK

This braid is a head-turner. By combining French braiding techniques with the fishtail braid style, you'll create a stunning herringbone-shaped braid. Once you've mastered the regular fishtail braid, you'll love adding the dynamic herringbone shape to your look. Best suited to long hair or hair without layers, this distinctive braid can be worn straight or curved into a chignon.

DIFFICULTY LEVEL
Hard

IDEAL HAIR LENGTH
Long

HAIR EXTENSIONS NEEDED?
No

ASSISTANCE NEEDED?
Yes

ACCESSORIES
With so much beautiful detail, this hairstyle doesn't need many accessories, but you can wear a headband to add a pretty touch to the front.

TRY THIS
By braiding your hair on a diagonal angle, you can create a beautiful side French fishtail braid. Curve your braid around to form a fishtail chignon.

▶ **SEE ALSO**
Fishtail braid, pages 32–33
Fishtail chignon,
pages 82–83

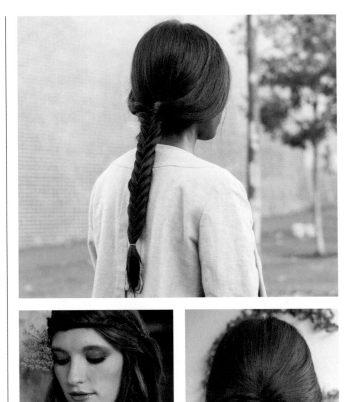

Top: Hairstyling by Christina Butcher, photography by Xiaohan Shen, modeling by Deauvanné.
Bottom left: Hairstyling and makeup by Erin Skipley, photography by Jasmine Star, modeling by Amber Anderson.
Bottom right: Hairstyling and photography by Christina Butcher, modeling by Carolyn Mach.

HOW TO GET IT

WHAT YOU NEED

- Brush
- Hair elastic

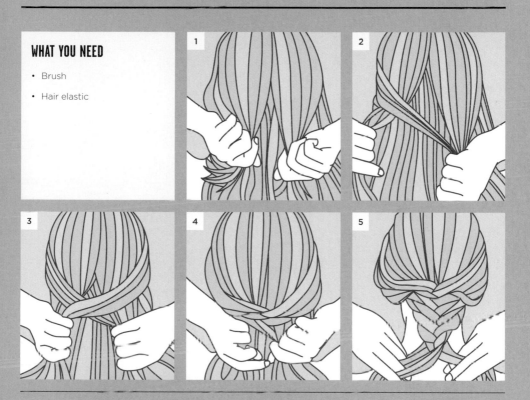

1. Brush your hair to remove any knots. Take a section of hair at the back of your head and split it into two equal sections.

2. Holding one section in each hand, use your index finger to add in hair from the left side of your head and cross it over and add to the right section.

3. Repeat this on the right side, picking up hair and adding it to the left section.

4. Continue adding in hair and crossing to the opposite section until there's no more hair left to add.

5. Finish in a regular fishtail braid and secure the end with an elastic.

TOP TIP

This style works best in long hair without too many layers. Try to keep each section small and even to emphasize the herringbone shape. You can also gently pull at the sides of the braid to give it more volume.

ROPE TWIST
THE LOOK

You've heard of a drink or a story with a twist—well, this is a style with the sweetest twist of all! The rope twist is a classic braid that can be worn on its own or used to add volume to buns and chignons. This simple two-strand braid holds itself together and gives the impression of being a much more complicated style.

DIFFICULTY LEVEL
Medium

IDEAL HAIR LENGTH
Long

HAIR EXTENSIONS NEEDED?
No, but you can use a ponytail extension in short hair.

ASSISTANCE NEEDED?
No

ACCESSORIES
Incorporate a ribbon or scarf into the twist to add some colorful detail: tie around the top of your ponytail and twist the ribbon or scarf in with your rope braid.

TRY THIS
Combine this with a side ponytail for a pretty variation or turn your rope twist into a top knot or low bun.

▶ **SEE ALSO**
Gibson roll, pages 68–69
Coiled bun, pages 76–77

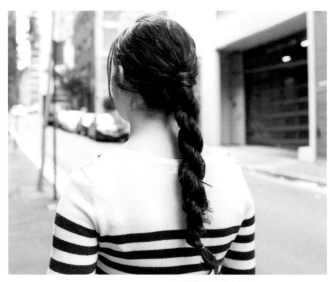

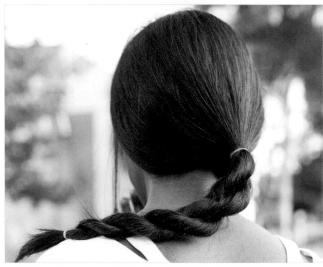

Top: Hairstyling by Christina Butcher, photography by Xiaohan Shen, modeling by Monica Bowerman .
Bottom: Hairstyling by Christina Butcher, photography by Xiaohan Shen, modeling by Deauvanné .

HOW TO GET IT

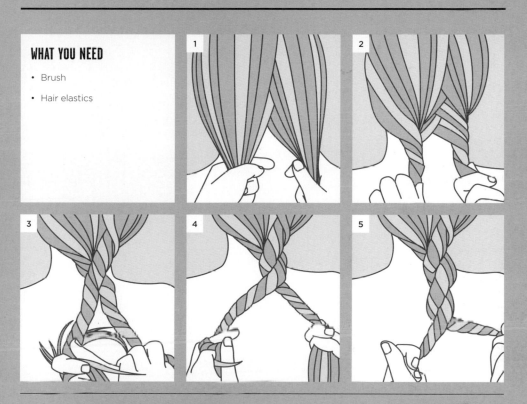

WHAT YOU NEED

- Brush
- Hair elastics

1. Brush your hair to remove any knots and split into two equal sections.
2. Twist each section to the right.
3. Cross the right section of hair over the left section to begin forming the rope twist.
4. Keep twisting the sections to the right and wrapping them to the left.
5. Secure the end of your braid with an elastic.

TOP TIP

Keep twisting the sections to the right so that they keep their shape as you wrap them together. You'll know if you have gone in the wrong direction if the braid falls flat. You can gently stretch out the sides of the braid to make your hair appear thicker.

HALF-UP HEART BRAID
THE LOOK

Wear your heart in your hair with this romantic braid, a clear favorite for a anniversary or Valentine's Day dinner. Braiding shapes into your hair can be great fun, and they add an extra dimension to braided styles. After you've mastered this heart shape, why not try some ideas of your own?

DIFFICULTY LEVEL
Medium

IDEAL HAIR LENGTH
Medium to long

HAIR EXTENSIONS NEEDED?
No

ASSISTANCE NEEDED?
Yes, but you can do this in your own hair with practice.

ACCESSORIES
Your hair forms the focus in this hairstyle, so no adornments are needed.

TRY THIS
You can create a heart in your hair wherever you can make two braids, such as at the side of your head. This hairstyle also looks great when you braid two hearts next to each other.

▶ **SEE ALSO**
Heart-shaped angel braid, pages 40–41
Grecian braid, pages 46–47

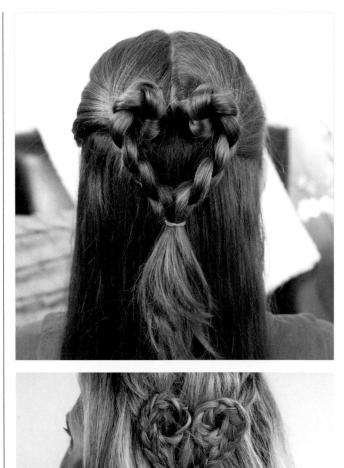

Top: Hairstyling, photography, and modeling by Mindy McKnight.
Bottom: Hairstyling, photography, and modeling by Christina Butcher.

HOW TO GET IT

WHAT YOU NEED

- Brush
- Small clear hair elastics
- Bobby pins

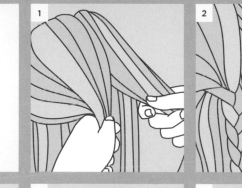

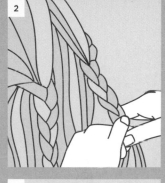

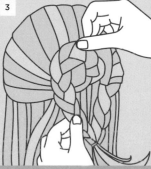

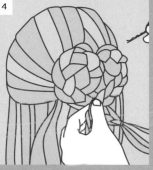

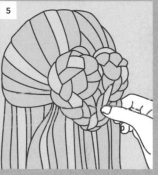

1. Brush your hair and section off the top half of your hair. Split into two equal sections.

2. Braid each section using the basic braid technique and secure the ends with small clear elastics.

3. Loop the left-hand braid up and around to form the top of the heart. Pin in place with bobby pins.

4. Repeat with the right-hand braid, coiling it around to form the top of the heart. Use bobby pins to secure it in place.

5. You can finish either in a ponytail by removing the elastics from the ends of each braid and securing them together with one elastic, or by folding the tails of each braid up to form the point of the heart. Tuck in any loose ends and pin in place with bobby pins.

TOP TIP

Use clear elastics or elastics that match your hair color, as they will be less conspicuous in the heart shape. If you have very long hair, the braids can be folded in half before forming the heart.

WATERFALL BRAID
THE LOOK

This style uses the French braiding technique, however instead of picking up a new section of hair from the bottom, you allow it to flow through, creating a cascading waterfall effect. This braid can be done in any length of hair. The stunning waterfall braid is perfect for long days on the beach and casual outdoor parties and is a gorgeous choice for the boho bride. It takes some practice but looks fabulous when you get it right!

DIFFICULTY LEVEL
Hard

IDEAL HAIR LENGTH
Any

HAIR EXTENSIONS NEEDED?
No

ASSISTANCE NEEDED?
Yes, but you can do this in your own hair with practice.

ACCESSORIES
The beauty of this braid lies in the elegant falling sections, so you don't have to decorate this style further. For a sweet touch you could finish the braid off with a simple ribbon or weave a daisy chain through the waterfall.

TRY THIS
You can start from the left and work right, depending on which side you prefer to part your hair. This braid forms part of the water-fall bun and can be doubled up to form a double waterfall braid.

▶ **SEE ALSO**
Angel braid, pages 30–31
Twist-over ponytail, pages 16–17

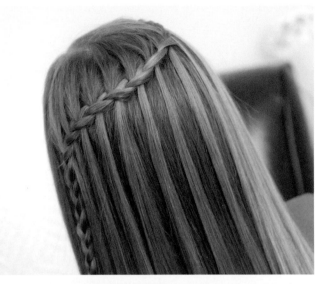

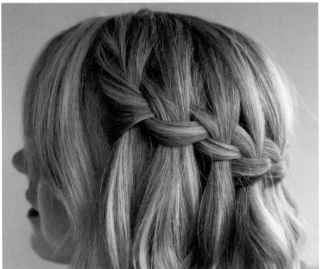

Top: Hairstyling, photography, and modeling by Mindy McKnight.
Bottom: Hairstyling, photography, and modeling by Christina Butcher.

HOW TO GET IT

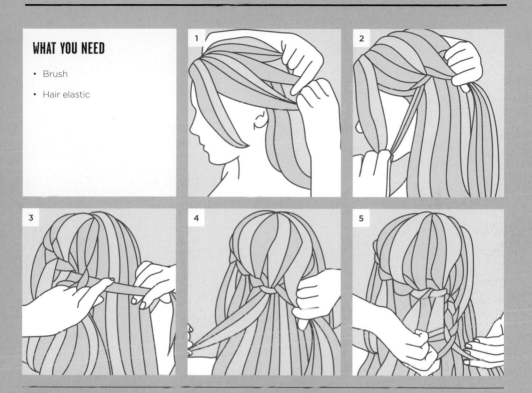

WHAT YOU NEED

- Brush
- Hair elastic

1. Brush all of your hair back and away from your face. If you have bangs, you can leave them out. To start, take a 1- to 2-inch section of hair from the left side of your head and split it into three equal parts.

2. Begin braiding by crossing section 1 over 2 and then section 3 over 1. Add in hair from the top of your head to section 2 and then cross it over section 3.

3. Next, instead of crossing section 1 over 2, drop it out and pick up a new piece of hair from just behind it. Cross this over section 2 and continue braiding.

4. Only add in hair from the top, and drop out the bottom piece as you go, remembering to pick up a new piece from behind it.

5. When you reach the right side, stop adding in hair, finish off the waterfall braid, and secure with an elastic (see the Top Tip for finishing ideas).

TOP TIP

There are two ways to finish off your waterfall braid: in a regular braid or in a loose ponytail. Reach your arm right over your head when you start, and every time you grab a section of hair, add it to the braid, let it drop, and replace it with a new section.

LACE BRAID
THE LOOK

The lace braid is a half French braid with a delicate scalloped edge. By brushing your hair forward you can create a braided layer of hair that frames your face. The way the long sections come down to meet the braid on your hairline makes this style look like an upside-down waterfall braid.

DIFFICULTY LEVEL
Medium

IDEAL HAIR LENGTH
Medium to long

HAIR EXTENSIONS NEEDED?
No

ASSISTANCE NEEDED?
Yes, but you can do this in your own hair with practice.

ACCESSORIES
You could weave a fine ribbon through the braid to give the style an extra accent of pretty! Finish the braid with a small bow or decorative band.

TRY THIS
This braid looks beautiful if you start with a center part and mirror the braid on both sides around your face.

▶ **SEE ALSO**
Angel braid, pages 30–31
Waterfall braid, pages 58–59

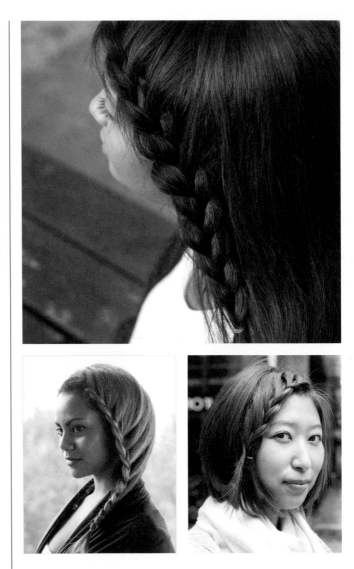

Top: Hairstyling and photography by Christina Butcher, modeling by Nicole Jeyaraj.
Bottom left: Hairstyling and photography by Christina Butcher, modeling by Dorothy Jean Joly.
Bottom right: Hairstyling by Christina Butcher, photography by Xiaohan Shen, modeling by Hitomi Nakajima.

HOW TO GET IT

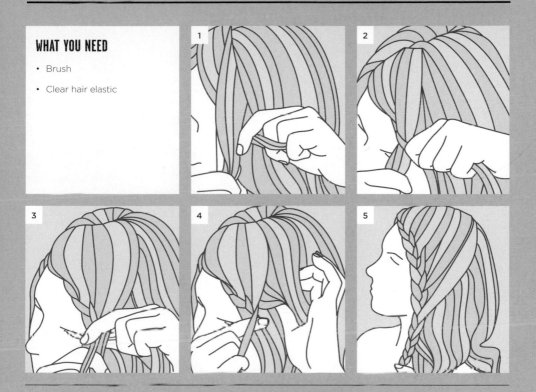

WHAT YOU NEED

- Brush
- Clear hair elastic

1. Brush your hair and make a deep side part on the right side of your head. Take a small section of hair at the start of the part and split it into three.

2. Start the French braid here, but only add in hair from behind (not from your hairline).

3-4. Keep adding in very small sections to your braid until you reach your cheekbone or jaw line.

5. Finish in a regular braid and secure with a clear elastic.

TOP TIP

Angle the braid right onto your face and in front of your hairline. You want the braid to sit grazing the edge of your eyebrow and come down the left side of your face.

PRETZEL BRAID
THE LOOK

This pretty twist on pigtails is a fun way to wear your hair up. Two pigtail braids twist around each other in a pretzel shape that sits low at the back of your head. This style doesn't have to be precise—the idea is to create a nice curved shape from the braid. The look is cool, modern, and distinctive and complements any outfit.

DIFFICULTY LEVEL
Medium

IDEAL HAIR LENGTH
Long

HAIR EXTENSIONS NEEDED?
No

ASSISTANCE NEEDED?
Yes, but you can do this in your own hair with practice.

ACCESSORIES
Because this is a decorative braid, you don't want to overdo it with more accessories. A simple pin at the center draws attention to your braid.

TRY THIS
Once you've mastered this version, try creating other shapes and styles with your pigtails. You can also try the pretzel style using the fishtail braid (see pages 32-33).

▶ **SEE ALSO**
Coiled bun, pages 76-77
Braided side bun, pages 80-81

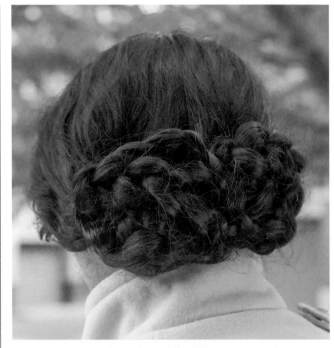

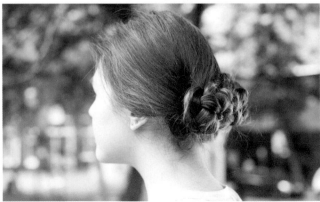

Top: Hairstyling and photography by Christina Butcher, modeling by Tanu Vasu.
Bottom: Hairstyling by Christina Butcher, photography by Xiaohan Shen, modeling by Sophia Phan.

HOW TO GET IT

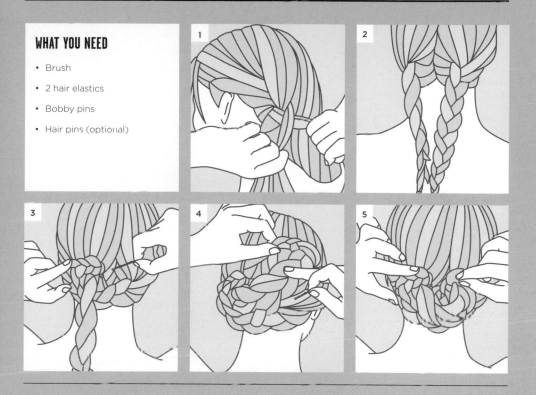

WHAT YOU NEED

- Brush
- 2 hair elastics
- Bobby pins
- Hair pins (optional)

1. Brush your hair and split it down the middle into two equal sections.

2. Braid both sections into pigtails and secure the ends with elastics.

3. Cross one braid over the other. Take the braid that's now below and twist it around the other braid to create a "C" shape. Pin in place with bobby pins.

4. Repeat with the other braid, curving it up and around to make the same shape, and pin in place.

5. Adjust your braids to sit in a kind of pretzel or knot shape at the back of your head. Tuck the ends of your braids behind the knot and pin them using bobby pins. Use hairpins to secure the style if you have thick hair.

TOP TIP

Start your pigtails a little higher on your head so that you have more space to arrange your pretzel-shaped bun. If you need help keeping your braids in place, you can section your hair with elastics before braiding, but remember to remove them before assembling the pretzel shape.

TOP KNOT BUN
THE LOOK

So French, so chic! The top knot is an effortless hairstyle that always looks stylish. It's easy to do and a good way to hide less-than-perfect hair while still maintaining some fashion cred. The cool top knot sits high on the crown of your head, adding height to your look. The top knot looks and holds best in second-day hair.

DIFFICULTY LEVEL
Easy

IDEAL HAIR LENGTH
Long

HAIR EXTENSIONS NEEDED?
No

ASSISTANCE NEEDED?
No

ACCESSORIES
Top knot buns are a great base for all kinds of accessories. Headbands add instant detail to the front, and you can add flowers, scarves, or bows to accessorize the back.

TRY THIS
Wear it messy for an effortless look, or try one of the variations in this chapter for extra detail. The donut bun or braided bun are great examples.

▶ **SEE ALSO**
Figure-8 bun, pages 72–73
Coiled bun, pages 76–77

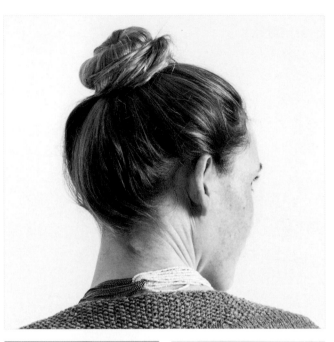

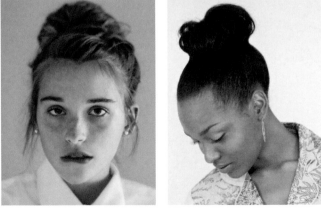

Top: Photograph courtesy of Brooklyn Tweed. Hairstyling by Stephanie Gelot and Aine Vonnegut, photography by Jared Flood, modeling by Aine Vonnegut.
Bottom left: Hairstyling, photography, and modeling by Alison Titus.
Bottom right: Photograph courtesy of Plum Pretty Sugar. Hairstyling by Makeup 1011 and Katie M, photography by Marisa Holmes.

HOW TO GET IT

WHAT YOU NEED

- Brush
- Hair elastic
- Bobby pins or hairpins
- Hairspray (optional)

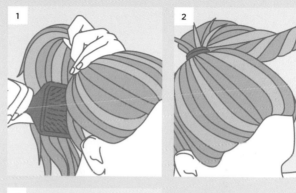

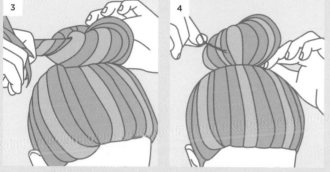

1. Brush your hair and gather it up into a high ponytail. Secure with a strong elastic.

2. Loosely twist your hair and then loop it around the base of the ponytail. If you have long hair, you may need to loop it around twice, but don't pull your hair too tight, because you want the bun to be a little loose.

3. Secure the base of the bun with bobby pins or hairpins.

4. If required, finish with a spritz of hairspray to hold any flyaways and loose pieces of hair.

TOP TIP

All you need to secure your bun is four bobby pins—one at both the front and back and one at each side. For thick hair try using hairpins instead. Don't be too precise with top knots —they can give you a headache if they're too tight, and you want it to look effortless.

FISHTAIL BRAIDED BUN
THE LOOK

Amp up the texture in your top knot with this fishtail braided bun. This hairstyle works best in long hair, but you can use extensions or padding to add more volume to the finished look. The braid is made up of two fishtail braids that twist around to form a top knot. You can't really tell that it's a fishtail braid when it's finished, but you can see the beautiful herringbone texture of the braid. Fishtail braids are traditionally messy, so be prepared for the bun to be messy too. This is an excellent look for a day out with friends.

DIFFICULTY LEVEL
Medium

IDEAL HAIR LENGTH
Long

HAIR EXTENSIONS NEEDED?
No

ASSISTANCE NEEDED?
Yes

ACCESSORIES
With so much detail in the fishtail braided bun, you can keep it simple with your hair accessories. A classic barrette or headband is all that's needed to dress up this hairstyle.

TRY THIS
If you have very long hair, you can just do one braid and wind it all the way around to form the bun. Alternatively, try braiding three or four smaller fishtail braids and twist them up into a more detailed bun.

▶ **SEE ALSO**
Fishtail braid, pages 32–33
Braided side bun, pages 80–81

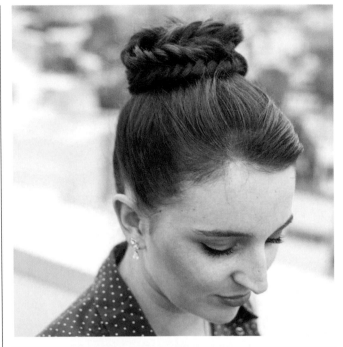

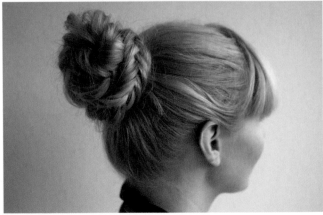

Top: Hairstyling and photography by Christina Butcher, modeling by Elly Hanson.
Bottom: Hairstyling and photography by Christina Butcher, modeling by Michaela Williams.

HOW TO GET IT

WHAT YOU NEED

- Paddle brush or bristle brush
- Strong hair elastic
- Hair clip
- 2 small clear hair elastics
- Bobby pins

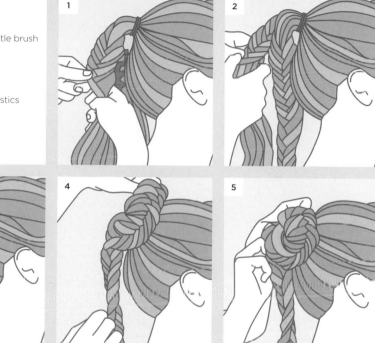

1. Brush your hair using a paddle or bristle brush and gather it into a high ponytail. Secure with a strong hair elastic.

2. Split your ponytail in two and clip away one half. Split the other section in two and begin to fishtail braid (see pages 32–33). Secure the end of the braid with a small clear elastic. Repeat, fishtail braiding the other half of your ponytail.

3. Stretch out your fishtail braids.

4. Take the first braid and twist it up and around the base of your ponytail and pin in place with bobby pins.

5. Repeat step 4 with the second braid, twisting in the opposite direction to create a full bun. Secure the bun with bobby pins.

TOP TIP

Stretching out your braids before twisting them into the bun emphasizes the delicate shape of the braids and adds more detail to the finished bun. You can still adjust the bun once it is pinned in place, but it's easier to shape the braids beforehand.

GIBSON ROLL
THE LOOK

The Gibson roll is an elegant twisted upstyle that's perfect for more formal events. This classic style became popular in the 1940s, and this version is a modern twist on the original design. Start with a ponytail and simply roll your hair into a space above it. Gibson rolls are surprisingly simple to do and create an elegant silhouette, with the roll curving around from the back of your neck.

DIFFICULTY LEVEL
Medium

IDEAL HAIR LENGTH
Medium to long

HAIR EXTENSIONS NEEDED?
No

ASSISTANCE NEEDED?
No

ACCESSORIES
This sophisticated hairstyle creates the perfect space for accessories. Add your favorite jewels to the top of the roll to create a refined formal updo. Fresh or silk flowers are also perfect in this chic upstyle.

TRY THIS
You can create a more asymmetrical look by tucking your hair into the Gibson roll off to one side. Create more detail at the sides by leaving the front sections of your hair loose and twisting them back into the top of the Gibson roll.

▶ **SEE ALSO**
Pretzel braid, pages 62–63
Gibson roll, pages 68–69

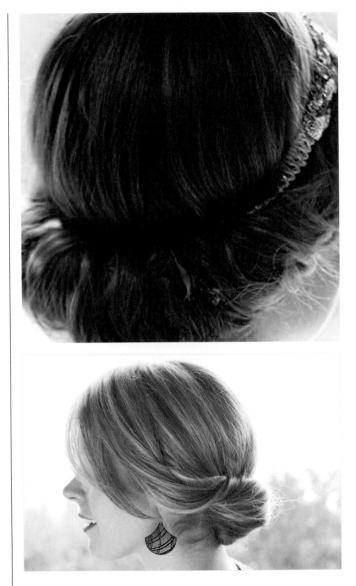

Top: Hairstyling, photography, and modeling by Lana Red Studio.
Bottom: Hairstyling and modeling by Christina Butcher, photography by Xiaohan Shen.

HOW TO GET IT

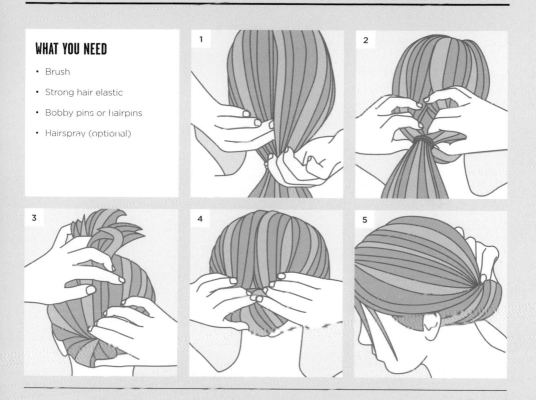

WHAT YOU NEED

- Brush
- Strong hair elastic
- Bobby pins or hairpins
- Hairspray (optional)

1. Brush your hair and gather it into a ponytail that sits low at the back of your head. Secure in place with a strong hair elastic.

2. Next, slide the hair elastic 1 to 2 inches down your ponytail so that you create a space between your hair elastic and your scalp.

3. Push your fingers in above your hair elastic to make a gap. Don't push all the way through; just create a space inside that can hold your hair.

4. Twist your ponytail up and begin pushing it down into this little space. Continue tucking and rolling your ponytail into the gap.

5. Once you have all your hair hidden and tucked away, pin it in place with bobby pins or hairpins. Finish with a spritz of hairspray to hold this hairstyle all day and all night!

TOP TIP

Don't forget to pin the sides of your hair into the roll as well. When you first begin tucking your hair into the space above your ponytail, it may seem tight, but keep twisting your hair to create the roll shape.

FRENCH TWIST
THE LOOK

This classic style has been worn by style icons for generations. The French twist, roll, or pleat is a chic updo that's as easy as twist and pin! The French twist is a sophisticated hairstyle that works from day to night.

DIFFICULTY LEVEL
Medium

IDEAL HAIR LENGTH
Medium to long

HAIR EXTENSIONS NEEDED?
No

ASSISTANCE NEEDED?
Yes, but you can do this style in your own hair with practice.

ACCESSORIES
The side of the French twist can take any accessory to match your outfit. Try jeweled pins or pin fresh or silk flowers to add a bohemian twist.

TRY THIS
This sophisticated style can be worn sleek and smooth for an elegant evening style, or left loose and messy for a chic daytime style. The French twist is normally worn straight up the back of your head, but it can also be swept to the side for an asymmetrical twist.

▶ **SEE ALSO**
French braid, pages 24–25
Classic 1960s bouffant, pages 86–87

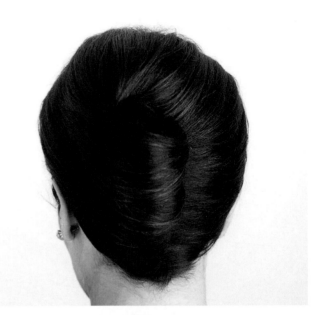

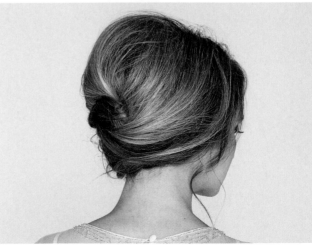

Top: Hairstyling by Ky Wilson/Electric Hairdressing London, photography by Matt Jones Photography.
Bottom: Hairstyling and modeling by Jordan Byers, photography by Tec Petaja.

HOW TO GET IT

WHAT YOU NEED

- Brush
- Bobby pins
- Hairpins (optional)

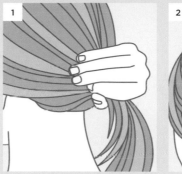

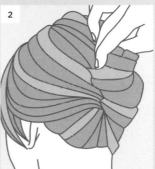

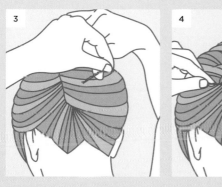

1. Brush your hair and gather it into a low ponytail.

2. Twist the length of your ponytail down and then flip it vertically up.

3. Fold the end of your ponytail over and tuck the ends inside to form a roll.

4. Pin the edge of the twist in place with bobby pins. If you have thick hair, use hairpins for a stronger, more secure finish.

TOP TIP

To keep the French twist in place, angle your bobby pins horizontally. For a secure finish, pin from left to right, twisting the pin 180 degrees so that you catch hair from the top of the twist, and then push the pin underneath the twist.

FIGURE-8 BUN
THE LOOK

The figure-8 bun is, quite literally, a clever twist on the traditional bun. Twisting the hair into a bun and then twisting out the center creates an 8-shaped bun that will set your hairstyle apart from the rest. This is a very neat style that suits professional settings and smart events.

DIFFICULTY LEVEL
Medium

IDEAL HAIR LENGTH
Long

HAIR EXTENSIONS NEEDED?
Yes, this style is best in long to very long hair.

ASSISTANCE NEEDED?
No

ACCESSORIES
Push a decorative hair stick down through the center of the bun to add a little Far Eastern flair to the style.

TRY THIS
Wear your bun sideways and turn it into an infinity bun!

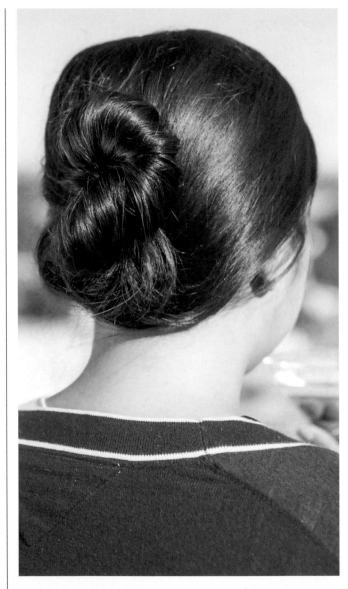

▶ **SEE ALSO**
Bobble ponytail, pages 20–21
Figure-8 braid, pages 44–45

Hairstyling and photography by Christina Butcher, modeling by An Ly.

HOW TO GET IT

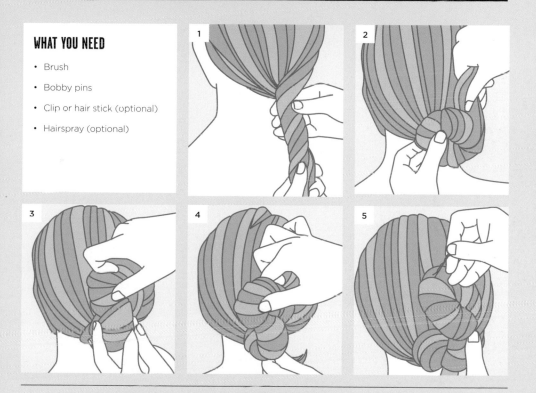

WHAT YOU NEED

- Brush
- Bobby pins
- Clip or hair stick (optional)
- Hairspray (optional)

1. Brush your hair into a low ponytail and twist it down. If you're right-handed, twist counter-clockwise, and if you're left-handed, twist clockwise.

2. Keep twisting your hair around and into a low bun.

3. Take the center part of your bun (the first twist-around) and flip it up and above your original bun.

4. Adjust the twist to sit in a flat figure-8 shape. Ensure the ends are tucked in at the base or side of your bun, depending on how long your hair is.

5. Secure the figure-8 bun with bobby pins at the top and base. You can also insert a hair stick vertically through the center or use a clip across the center to keep this style in place. If needed, use a spritz of hairspray for extra hold.

TOP TIP

Keep the twist tight (but not too tight!) to help maintain the shape and sleekness of this unique bun.

UPSIDE-DOWN BRAID BUN
THE LOOK

Named after its structure, the upside-down braid bun begins as a braid at your neckline and works its way up to a bun at your crown. This style ticks all the boxes in one go: not only does it combine a beautiful braid with a neat, functional bun, it also adds height to your hair and allows for variation. For that reason, this style is great for all occasions, formal, informal, at home, or away on vacation.

DIFFICULTY LEVEL
Hard

IDEAL HAIR LENGTH
Medium to long

HAIR EXTENSIONS NEEDED?
No, but extensions can be used if you want a big bun to finish.

ASSISTANCE NEEDED?
Yes. The tutorial shows you how to do it in your own hair, but this style is easiest with a partner.

ACCESSORIES
There's a lot going on with this hairstyle, so you really don't need to add anything to it.

TRY THIS
There are so many ways to customize this hairstyle. Try a French braid instead of a Dutch braid at the back. You could even try a French fishtail braid in long hair. Then there's the bun: try a donut bun, a messy bun, or a braided bun!

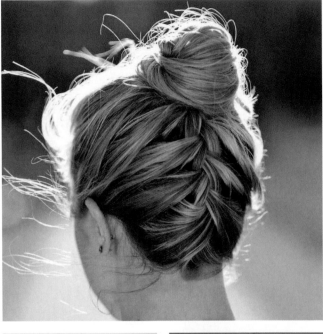

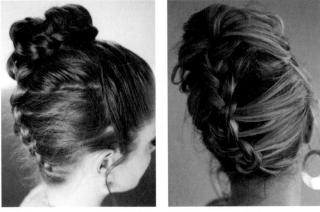

▶ **SEE ALSO**
French braid, pages 24–25
Braided side bun, pages 80–81

Top: Hairstyling, modeling, and photography by Kayley Heeringa.
Bottom left: Hairstyling by Ceci Meyer/Tribe Hair Studio, photography by Brittany Lauren Photography.
Bottom right: Hairstyling, photography, and modeling by Christina Butcher.

HOW TO GET IT

WHAT YOU NEED

- Brush
- Hair clip
- Hair donut
  (optional—for donut bun)
- Bobby pins

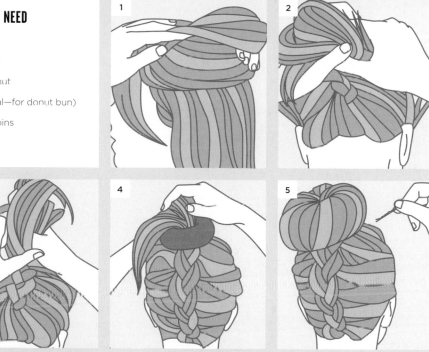

1. Brush your hair and clip up the top section of hair above your crown.

2. Hang your head down, ready to begin the braid from the nape of your neck. Take a 1-inch section at your hairline, split it into three, and start to Dutch braid (see pages 26–27).

3. With your head still down, continue braiding in a straight line up the back of your head toward your crown.

4. When you reach your crown, unclip the top section of hair and combine it with your braid in a high ponytail. If you're using a hair donut, place this at the base of your ponytail.

5. Hide the donut by twisting and wrapping your hair around it. If you have long hair, simply twist your hair around into a top knot and pin in place with bobby pins.

TOP TIP

When your braid reaches the crown of your head, finish in a basic braid so that it stays in place and is easier to combine with the rest of your hair.

COILED BUN
THE LOOK

Inspired by the Topsy Tail hair tool, this style creates an intricate mess of twists and swirls in a bun that sits low on your head or at your neckline. The process of turning the hair inside itself over and over gives the impression of many buns combined into one. This style can be made to look as messy or as neat as you'd like.

DIFFICULTY LEVEL
Medium

IDEAL HAIR LENGTH
Long

HAIR EXTENSIONS NEEDED?
Yes, you can use extensions for short or fine hair.

ASSISTANCE NEEDED?
No

ACCESSORIES
You can add a clip or flower to the top of the coiled bun. Aside from adding an accessory, this will also help disguise the part at the top of your bun.

TRY THIS
For a different result, try pulling the end of your ponytail through the hole from underneath instead of going up and over. It's slightly more difficult, but it creates a great effect.

▶ **SEE ALSO**

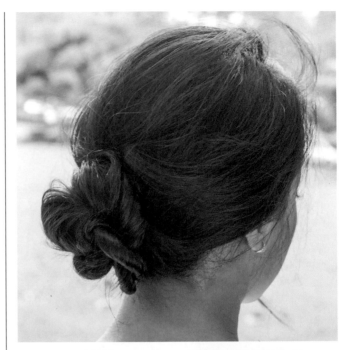

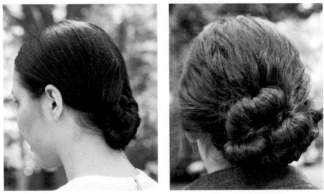

Top: Hairstyling and photography by Christina Butcher, modeling by Patricia Almario.
Bottom left: Hairstyling by Christina Butcher, photography by Xiaohan Shen, modeling by Tash Williams.
Bottom right: Hairstyling by Christina Butcher, photography by Xiaohan Shen, modeling by Monica Bowerman.

HOW TO GET IT

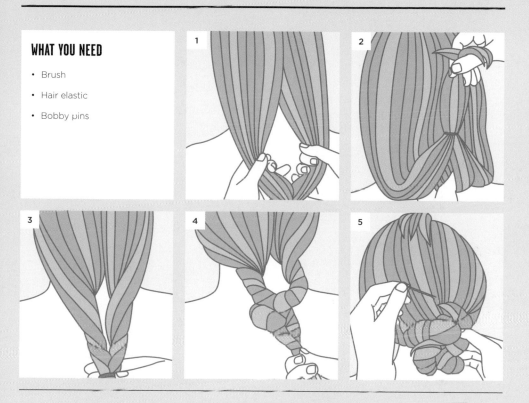

WHAT YOU NEED

- Brush
- Hair elastic
- Bobby pins

1. Brush your hair back into a low ponytail and secure with a hair elastic. Slide the hair elastic down your ponytail, leaving 2 to 3 inches of hair at the end.

2. Split your hair in the middle above your hair elastic and flip your hair up, over, and through the hole above your ponytail.

3. Repeat step 2, flipping your hair through the hole, and you'll see your hair starting to coil and twist.

4. Continue flipping your hair until it coils tightly and forms a bun shape.

5. Tuck the ends of your ponytail underneath and hide them under the coils. Pin your bun in place with bobby pins.

TOP TIP

Make sure the elastic you use is tight enough to hold the end of your ponytail as you flip and twist. If it's not, your hair will come loose and you'll lose the texture you'll need to create this bun.

BOW BUN
THE LOOK

Lady Gaga loves this style, and it's no wonder, as there's a sense of living art about it. Turning your hair into something you usually accessorize with creates an intriguing look that not only mesmerizes, but is also super cute! This fun style is perfect for days when you're feeling whimsical and creative.

DIFFICULTY LEVEL
Medium

IDEAL HAIR LENGTH
Long

HAIR EXTENSIONS NEEDED?
No

ASSISTANCE NEEDED?
No

ACCESSORIES
Accessories aren't needed with this style, but wear with polka dots for the ultimate Minnie Mouse look!

TRY THIS
Make a bow bun with only half your hair for a more textured and relaxed feel, or wear the bun at the nape of your neck to produce a sleek look.

▶ **SEE ALSO**
Bow braids, pages 34–35
Heart-shaped angel braid, pages 40–41

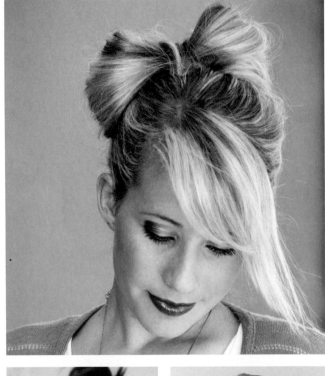

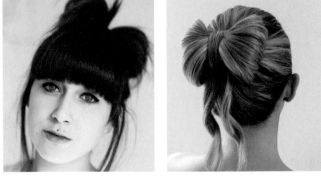

Top: Hairstyling, photography, and modeling by Abby Smith/Twist Me Pretty.
Bottom left: Hairstyling, photography, and modeling by Ana Santl.
Bottom right: Hairstyling, photography, and modeling by Jemma Grace.

HOW TO GET IT

WHAT YOU NEED

- Brush
- Strong hair elastic
- Bobby pins
- Hairspray (optional)

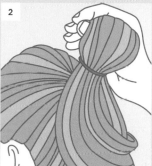

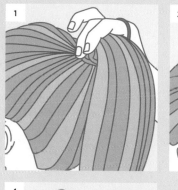

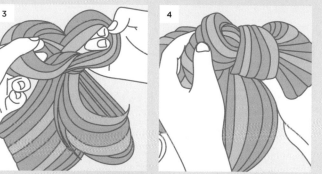

1. Brush your hair up into a high ponytail at the crown of your head. Use a strong hair elastic to secure in place.

2. On the final twist of your elastic, pull your hair only partway through, creating a loop in your ponytail.

3. Split the loop in two and pull each section out and to the side. This will form the sides of your hair bow.

4. Use the tail of your hair to form the center of the bow. Wrap it up and over the middle of the loop and use bobby pins to secure it at the front and back. Adjust the sides of the bow to sit evenly, and use bobby pins to keep them in place. A spritz of hairspray will smooth any flyaway hairs and fix the look.

TOP TIP

Use a bobby pin on either side of the tail that becomes the center ribbon of the bow to keep it straight and in place. If your hair is long, you can tuck the ends of your hair underneath so that they sit inside the loops of the bow.

BRAIDED SIDE BUN
THE LOOK

A simple donut bun can easily be transformed with a side braid detail. In this style a Dutch braid frames your face and wraps around your bun to create a chic look from every angle. The braided side bun can be messed up for a relaxed daytime feel or dressed up for a formal evening event. This type of hairstyle is especially perfect for parties, as you know it's going to last all night.

DIFFICULTY LEVEL
Medium

IDEAL HAIR LENGTH
Long

HAIR EXTENSIONS NEEDED?
No

ASSISTANCE NEEDED?
Yes, but you can do this style in your own hair with practice.

ACCESSORIES
The braid is the accessory in this style, although a sparkly pin or flower corsage would sit beautifully with this bun.

TRY THIS
If you've yet to master the Dutch braid (see pages 26–27), you can do a regular braid and wrap this around the bun to achieve a similar look. If your hair is very long, you can skip the donut bun and just twist your hair into a sleek bun at the side.

▶ **SEE ALSO**
   Fishtail braid, pages 32–33
   Fishtail chignon, pages 82–83

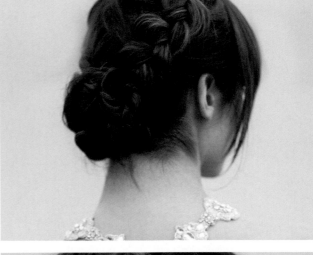

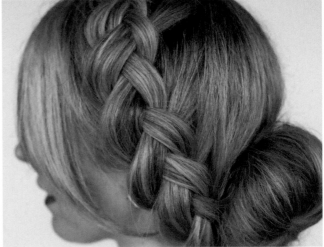

Top: Hairstyling and makeup by Amber Rose, photography by Autumn Wilson Photography, modeling by Laura.
Bottom: Hairstyling, photography, and modeling by Christina Butcher.

HOW TO GET IT

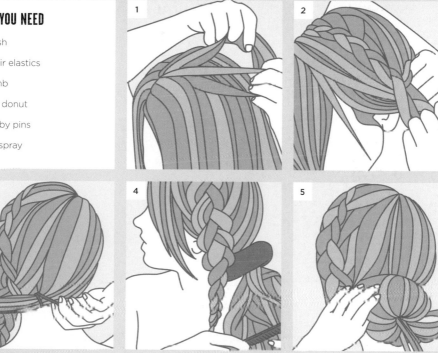

WHAT YOU NEED

- Brush
- 2 hair elastics
- Comb
- Hair donut
- Bobby pins
- Hairspray

1. Start by making a deep side part and brush your hair to remove any knots. Take a 1-inch section on top of your part and split it into three sections. This is the start of the Dutch braid.

2. Cross the right piece under the middle, then the left under the right. When you cross the middle section under, add in some hair.

3. Continue braiding, only adding in hair on the right-hand side. Angle your braid along your hairline and over the top of your ear. Stop adding in hair when you pass your ear. Finish the braid and secure with a small clear elastic. Gather the rest of your hair into a side ponytail, next to your braid, and secure with a hair elastic.

4. Backcomb your ponytail and use a hair donut at the base of your ponytail to create a large side bun.

5. Wrap your braid around the base of your bun and pin in place. Add a spritz of hairspray to finish the look.

TOP TIP

To achieve a big, dramatic braid, you'll need to gently pull at the sides to widen it. If you have bangs, you can leave them out or incorporate them. If you leave them out and then change your mind, you can easily pin them back underneath your braid.

FISHTAIL CHIGNON
THE LOOK

This is an interesting twist on the fishtail braid. Sometimes referred to as a seashell braid, this curving fishtail has a nice shell-like quality and is a lovely upstyle for day or night. This style is complicated and is one of the harder looks to master, but the effects are stunning and well worth the practice.

DIFFICULTY LEVEL
Hard

IDEAL HAIR LENGTH
Medium to long

HAIR EXTENSIONS NEEDED?
No

ASSISTANCE NEEDED?
Yes

ACCESSORIES
Jeweled pins or a beautiful brooch pinned into the chignon would certainly set this style on fire.

TRY THIS
If you have long hair, you can finish at step 5 and leave your hair out in a side fishtail braid. A simpler version is to do a regular fishtail braid and twist it up into a bun, or make it more complicated by doing a tighter braid and adding in another turn to the braid to create an S shape at the back of your head.

▶ **SEE ALSO**
French fishtail braid, pages 52–53
Fishtail braided bun, pages 66–67

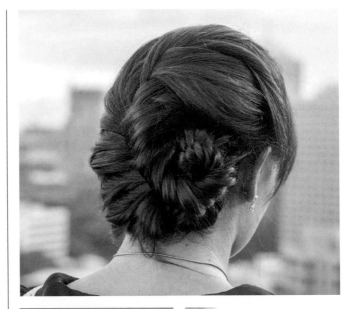

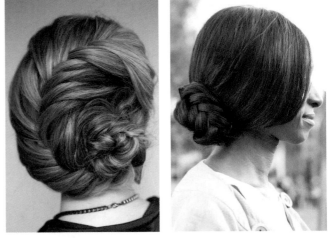

Top: Hairstyling and photography by Christina Butcher, modeling by Elly Hanson.
Bottom left: Hairstyling, photography, and modeling by Christina Butcher.
Bottom right: Hairstyling by Christina Butcher, photography by Xiaohan Shen, modeling by Deauvanné.

HOW TO GET IT

WHAT YOU NEED

- Brush
- Clear hair elastic
- Bobby pins
- Hairspray (optional)

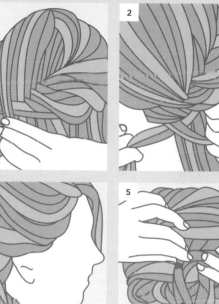

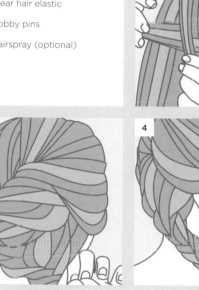

1. Brush your hair back and then make a short part on the right side of your head. Take a section of hair to begin your braid.

2. Make a French fishtail braid from top right to bottom left. French fishtail braids use the same technique as a regular fishtail, but you add in extra hair from each side as you braid. To do this, pick up a small section of hair from the left and cross it into your right hand, then pick up a small section of hair on the right and cross it over into your left hand. Repeat this as you braid diagonally downward.

3. When your braid reaches behind your left ear, start to curve it around and then braid along your lower hairline.

4. When you have reached the bottom right side of your head, continue into a regular side fishtail braid until all your hair is braided, and secure the end with a clear elastic.

5. Twist the braid up and around into a spiral bun. Pin in place with bobby pins and spritz some hairspray for extra hold.

TOP TIP

This hairstyle is best in long hair without too many layers. Try to keep each section you add in to the braid small and even. This will emphasize the seashell shape. See tips for mastering the French fishtail braid on pages 52-53.

MINI BUNS
THE LOOK

If you find the French twist difficult to master, this mini bun hairstyle is the perfect solution. The buns are easier to form without any assistance and will hold your hair well all day long. A row of mini buns down the back of your head in a straight line offers an elegant upstyle with a little edge that works from day to night.

DIFFICULTY LEVEL
Easy

IDEAL HAIR LENGTH
Medium

HAIR EXTENSIONS NEEDED?
No

ASSISTANCE NEEDED?
No

ACCESSORIES
You could pretty this hairstyle up with a jeweled pin, though this style doesn't require much adornment. A ribbon threaded around the buns and tied in a bow at the bottom would be a sweet touch.

TRY THIS
For long hair, braid each section before pinning it into a mini bun. You can do as many or as few buns as you like to suit your hair type.

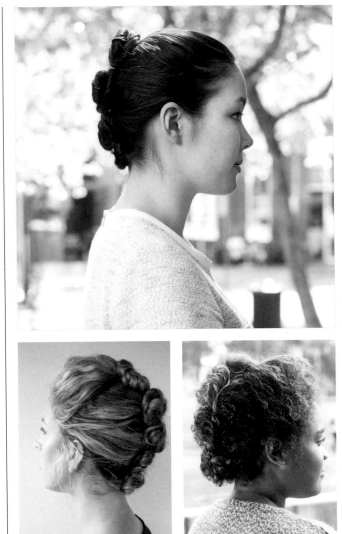

▶ SEE ALSO
  Twist-over ponytail,
  pages 16–17
  French twist, pages 70–71

Top: Hairstyling and photography by Christina Butcher, modeling by Tash Williams.
Bottom left: Hairstyling, photography, and modeling by Christina Butcher.
Bottom right: Hairstyling by Christina Butcher, photography by Xiaohan Shen, modeling by Ornella Joaquim.

HOW TO GET IT

WHAT YOU NEED

- Brush
- Bobby pins
- Hair elastics (optional, best for long/thick hair)

1. Brush your hair and pin back your bangs, or the front section of your hair, then secure with a bobby pin. This style looks good with a little height.

2. Take a small section from each side of your hairline and bring them together into a twist at the back of your head.

3. Twist the section around your finger and pin into a small bun. Secure with bobby pins.

4-5. Repeat steps 2 and 3 until all your hair is twisted and pinned into a line at the back of your head

TOP TIP

If you have thick or long hair, secure each section in a ponytail with a hair elastic before twisting into a mini bun.

CLASSIC 1960s BOUFFANT
THE LOOK

This is the most chic updo to come out of the 1960s. The beauty of this timeless classic is its stylish versatility. Perfect for a black-tie soirée or an important event, but also a great choice for work, this style's got it covered. Of course, the bouffant is best suited to the vintage '60s look, so think pencil skirts, simple straight dresses, and beautiful earrings. Also known as the beehive, this style originated in the 1950s and became iconic in the 1960s. Celebrities, notably Brigitte Bardot, favored the beehive style and made it extremely popular in the United States, where it was commonly styled using a fork!

DIFFICULTY LEVEL
Medium

IDEAL HAIR LENGTH
Medium to long

HAIR EXTENSIONS NEEDED?
Yes, the more hair the better for this style.

ASSISTANCE NEEDED?
No

ACCESSORIES
A wide satin headband is the perfect hair accessory to finish off the front of your bouffant. For an evening look, add a tiara!

TRY THIS
Leave this style relaxed and messy, with lots of volume at the top. You can modernize the bouffant with subtle volume, or wear your hair half down.

▶ **SEE ALSO**
1960s ponytail, pages 18–19
Gibson roll, pages 68–69

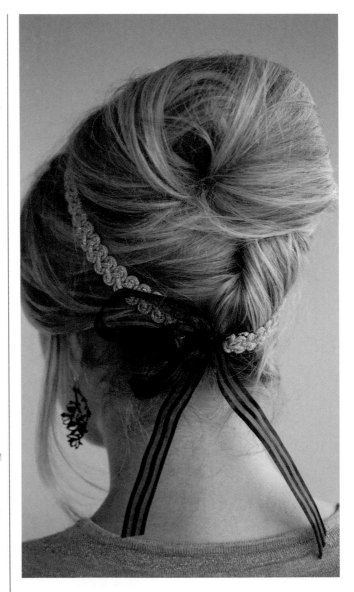

Hairstyling, photography, and modeling by Christina Butcher.

HOW TO GET IT

WHAT YOU NEED

- Hair clip
- Bobby pins or hairpins
- Comb
- Bristle brush
- Hairspray

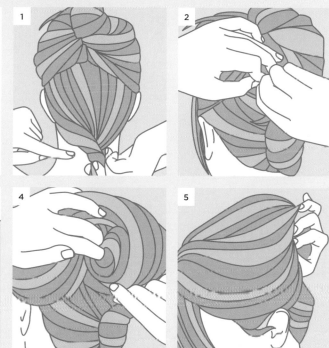

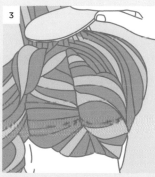

1. Part your hair from ear to ear at the back and clip the top section up. Take the bottom section of hair and twist it to the right into a low pony.

2. Flip your pony up and keep twisting your hair into a French twist (see pages 70–71). Tuck the ends of your hair inside the twist. Pin in place.

3. Backcomb the top section. Start at the crown and use a comb or fine bristle brush to tease your hair at the roots until it's almost standing up on its own. Use the fine bristle brush to smooth over the front layer.

4. Roll the ends of the top portion of hair around and under to form the base of your bouffant. Position it above the French twist and pin in place using bobby pins or hairpins.

5. Pin back the sides of your hair and make sure the top of your bouffant is smooth. If you have bangs, you can leave them loose or pin them back by your ear. Finish with lots of hairspray, just like they did in the 1960s. This will help your bouffant last all day and all night!

TOP TIP

To achieve huge volume in the bouffant, you'll need to use product to add structure and hold. If you have fine or soft hair, apply a volumizing mousse and use a blow dryer to set it into your hair. If your bouffant isn't holding, just keep backcombing and use more hairspray!

BEEHIVE WITH A BUN
THE LOOK

When the classic 1960s bouffant just isn't big enough, try a beehive with a bun. Using as much hair as possible is key to this style, and the hidden bun gives a more structured hold to the height of your beehive. You'll be ducking under doorways before you know it! This style still has the glamorous feel of the classic bouffant, just super-charged. This modern take on the beehive goes with my own motto: the higher the hair, the closer to heaven!

DIFFICULTY LEVEL
Hard

IDEAL HAIR LENGTH
Medium to long

HAIR EXTENSIONS NEEDED?
Yes, the more hair the better for this style.

ASSISTANCE NEEDED?
Yes, the tutorial offers a guide for doing this in your own hair, but it is much easier with help.

ACCESSORIES
An upstyle like this calls for statement earrings—the bigger the better.

TRY THIS
This hairstyle is itself a variation on the classic 1960s bouffant, and you can wear it with your hair half up for a more relaxed, messier upstyle.

SEE ALSO
French twist, pages 70–71
Classic 1960s bouffant, pages 86–87

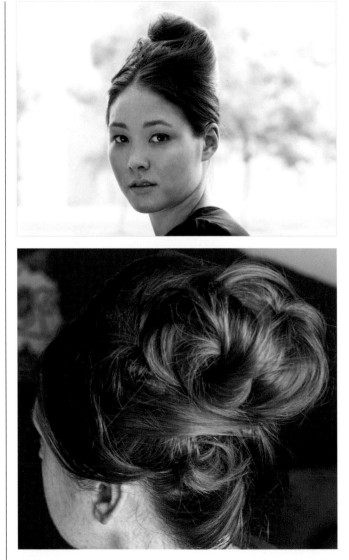

Top: Hairstyling by Christina Butcher, photography by Xiaohan Shen, modeling by Tash Williams.
Bottom: Hairstyling and photography by Christina Butcher, modeling by Monica Richmond.

HOW TO GET IT

WHAT YOU NEED

- Hair clip
- Comb
- Brush
- Bobby pins
- Hair elastic
- Hair donut
- Hairspray

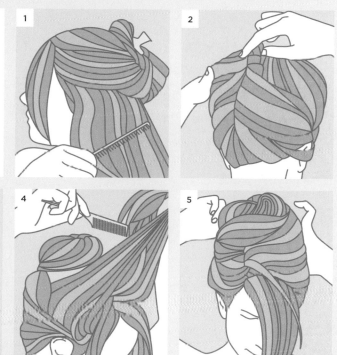

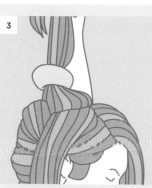

1. Separate your hair from ear to ear and clip the top section up. Use a comb to backcomb the bottom section of your hair at the roots.

2. Twist the bottom section down and then flip it up into a French twist (see pages 70–71). Brush the sides of your hair to smooth it back, tuck the ends of your hair inside the twist, and pin in place with bobby pins.

3. Take a 3-inch section of hair from the top at the crown, but make sure to leave enough hair at the front and sides for the later steps. Secure this section in a ponytail with a hair elastic and place the hair donut at the base. Backcomb your pony and cover the hair donut to create a bun.

4. Backcomb the rest of your loose hair. Focus on teasing at the roots and midlengths to create the shape and volume of the beehive.

5. Smooth the top of your hair and position your hair over and around the bun to create your beehive. Pin in place and use lots of hairspray. If you have bangs, you can leave them out or sweep them back.

TOP TIP

Visualize the style before you start to backcomb. Once the bun is in place, backcomb your hair with the shape in mind. This style adds extra lift, so you can get that wow factor with your super-high beehive even if you have fine or medium-length hair.

HAIRSTYLING TOOLS

Blow-dryer
A good blow-dryer is essential for your hairstyling kit. A professional dryer is best and will last a long time. Look for ionic blow-dryers, as this system reduces static and creates less frizz in your hair.

Conical curling iron
Barrel curlers have a set width, so always create the same sized curls. A conical curler allows you to create curls in different sizes and shapes, depending on where on the iron you heat-style your hair.

Curling iron
(with a clamp)
The original curling wand, which is designed to heat your hair to create curls and waves. The clamp helps you to hold your hair as you wind it around the barrel.

(without a clamp)
This newer type of curling wand is becoming increasingly popular. Use a heat-protective glove to protect your hand as you wind your hair around the barrel. This type of iron avoids the dents that a curling iron with a clamp can leave in your hair.

Diffuser
An attachment for your blow-dryer that disperses the air flow to spread it over a larger area. Use your dryer on a low speed with a diffuser to style curly hair.

Flat iron
Also known as straighteners or straightening irons, these heat-styling tools make your hair smooth and sleek. The ceramic plates glide down your hair, leaving it straighter than any blow-dryer can. You can also twist the iron through your hair to create waves.

Bristle brush
These brushes are best for smoothing your hair. They are made with boar bristles, which are gentler on hair than plastic brushes. The bristles also distribute your hair's natural oils and encourage shine.

Clips
Large clips are perfect for keeping sections of your hair out of the way while you are styling. Use the smaller flat clips to pin up curls when setting your hair.

Comb
Use the wide side to de-tangle wet hair and the fine side to backcomb for added height and volume.

Paddle brush
Great for detangling long hair. You can also use this brush when blow-drying, although it won't give as smooth a finish as a round brush.

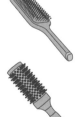

Round brush
Use a round brush to create volume and waves when blow-drying your hair. Wrap the ends of your hair around the brush to create flicks and waves, and use the cool-shot button on your blow-dryer to set the style.

Tail comb
Use the tail to section hair and create neat part lines. This fine comb is also great for backcombing and, used with straightening irons, will ensure there are no knots in your hair.

Bobby pins
The most important tool for any updo. Bobby pins are very handy, and you should always keep some in your bag. Choose pins that match your hair color, and look for professional pins, which are stronger than generic brands.

Fringe pins
These pins are fantastic for chignon and French twist styles, and even for securing braids in thick hair. The trick is to squeeze the pins a little when inserting them so that they spring into place and provide extra hold when you release them.

Hair bungees
Rather than pulling your hair through an elastic, hair bungees wrap around your hair. They are adjustable to suit hair thickness and are best for long hair, as they make it easier to secure ponytails. They are also curly-hair friendly—regular elastics can crush curls as you pull the hair through.

Hair donut
This round sponge padding is shaped like a donut and acts like a push up bra for your hair. It gives instant volume and shape to your bun. Hair donuts are available in different colors to match your hair. You can also make your own by cutting the toe off a sock and rolling it into a donut shape.

Hair elastics
Use to secure ponytails and braids as well as hair sections under buns. Find the right size and strength to hold your hair and look for snag-free elastics without metal connectors. Clear elastics are best for the ends of braids, as they are virtually invisible in your hair. Scrunchies should never be used!

Topsy Tail
This plastic tool works like a giant sewing needle for your hair. Place it above your hair elastic and thread your ponytail through the loop to neatly twist your hair back through itself. It's possible to re-create styles like the flipped-over ponytail (see pages 12–13) without it, but the Topsy Tail gives a neater finish.

Hairspray
The ultimate finishing spray for when you want your hairstyle to last. Don't overdo it with the hairspray though, as it can make your hair sticky and heavy. Choose a light, flexible hairspray when curling or backcombing your hair, and go for a strong-hold spray to fix an updo in place.

Serum
Serum smooths and adds shine to hair. It's available in tiny bottles, as you need only a drop or two to add gloss over your hair. Remember, a little goes a long way, and too much serum can make your hair look oily.

Styling powder
Styling powder adds instant volume. Lightly sprinkle these fine powders onto the roots of your hair and massage gently with your fingertips for an instant lift. These powders have a matte finish, so they can refresh oily roots.

GLOSSARY

Backcomb
Also known as teasing, ratting, matting, or French lacing. This technique involves combing small sections of hair from the ends toward the scalp, creating a cushion or base for hairstyles that require volume.

Bangs
Also known as a fringe, this is the front section of hair that falls across the face. You can style bangs in lots of ways—blunt bangs, curved bangs, or swept to the side. You can also leave them loose or include them in your hairstyles.

Blow-dry
Also called a blow-out. This is a styling technique where hair is dried and styled with a blow-dryer and usually with a round brush. You can also use a paddle brush when blow-drying long hair.

Braid
Also known as a plait. Chapter 2 in this book is devoted to this versatile styling technique, which involves winding or weaving sections of hair into each other.

Chignon
A twisted bun that usually sits low at the nape of your neck. The word "chignon" comes from the French phrase *chignon du cou*, which means "nape of the neck."

Crown
The area of the head along the top and back of the skull.

Curling iron/wand
A round- or conical-barrel heat styling tool that creates curls and waves.

Flat iron
A styling tool that straightens your hair. Also known as a straightening iron.

French plait
The same as a French braid.

Hair elastic
Used to tie up and secure hair. Also known as a hair band or tie.

Hair extensions
Hair that is attached to your natural hair to add length, volume, or texture. Extensions can be permanently attached or temporarily clipped in.

Hairline
This is the hair that grows along the outermost perimeters of your head, including around the face and ears and along the neck.

Hairspray
Also known as finishing spray, this is a styling product that comes in the form of a mist and is used to set a style in place.

Neckline
The neckline is part of the hairline, but specifically refers to the hair that begins at the back of the neck.

CONTRIBUTORS

Abby Smith, Twist Me Pretty
www.twistmepretty.com

Alison Titus
www.alison.titus.bz

Amber Rose Hair + Makeup
www.amberrosehairandmakeup.com

Photography: Eliesa Johnson Photography
www.eliesajohnson.com
Autumn Wilson Photography
www.autumnwilson.com

Wardrobe: Anne Kristine Lingerie
www.annekristinelingerie.com

Ana Santl
www.iamnotana.com

Breanna Rutter, How To Black Hair LLC
www.howtoblackhair.com

Brittany Lauren Photography
www.brittanylauren.net

Hairstyling: Ceci Meyer, Tribe Hair Studio
www.tribehairstudio.com

Brooklyn Tweed
www.brooklyntweed.net

Photography: Jared Flood, www.brooklyntweed.net
Hairstyling: Veronik Avery, www.stdenisyarns.com
Karen Schaupeter, www.karenschaupeter.com
Make-up: Hannah Metz, www.hannahkristinametz.co

Christina Butcher, Hair Romance
www.hairromance.com

Photography: Xiaohan Shen, www.xiaohan.com.au

Emily Goswick, The Rancher's Daughter
www.egoswick.blogspot.com

Emily M. Meyers, The Freckled Fox
www.freckled-fox.com

Erin Skipley
www.erinskipley.com

Photography: Elizabeth Messina
www.elizabethmessina.com
Jasmine Star, www.jasminestar.com

Fine Featherheads
www.finefeatherheads.com

Photography: Kate Broussard, Soulshots
Photography
www.soulshotsphoto.com

Jemma Grace
www.jemmagrace.com

Jordan Byers
www.jordanbyers.blogspot.com

Photography: Tec Petaja, www.tecpelajaphoto.com

Kayley Heeringa
www.sidewalkready.com

Photography: Kai Heeringa Photography
www.kaiheeringaphotography.com

Ky Wilson, Electric Hairdressing London
www.kycut.co.uk
www.electric-hair.com

Photography: Matt Jones Photography
mattjonesphoto.co.uk

Lana Red Studio
www.lanaredstudio.com

Marie-Pierre Sander
www.studiomariepierre.com

Mindy McKnight
www.cutegirlshairstyles.com

Plum Pretty Sugar
www.plumprettysugar.com

Hairstyling: Makeup 1011, www.1011makeup.com
Katie M, www.katiem.pixpasites.com
Photography: Marisa Holmes
www.marisaholmesblog.com

Suzy Wimbourne Photography
www.suzywimbourne.com

INDEX

ACKNOWLEDGMENTS

The following people have been instrumental in the making of this book, and without them there would be no way I could have possibly put *40 Ways to Style Your Hair* together.

First and foremost I should thank my husband, Jim, who has been my pillar of strength in the times when I didn't think I'd get this book finished. I also want to include my mum, Jeanette, and sister, Mary, for their constant help, advice, and support.

I want to thank Isheeta, at RotoVision, for her tireless patience throughout, and Diane, my editor, whose constructive criticism has helped make this book so very good. Also, the book's picture researcher, Heidi; Xiaohan, my photographer; and, of course, all of my hair models:

Abigail Schiavello, Adeline Er, An Ly, Arisa Nokubo, Ashleigh Forster, Barbara Rainbird, Carolyn Mach, Delphine Peyriere, Deauvanné, Dorothy Jean Joly, Elly Hanson, Emily Yeo, Hitomi Nakajima, Jane Proust, Jessica Schild, Jessica Tran, Laura Muheim, Michaela Williams, Monica Bowerman, Monica Richmond, Nicole Jeyaraj, Nina Lutz, Olivia English, Ornella Joaquim , Patricia Almario, Riko Ishihata, Ruri Okubo, Sam Colden, Sinead Brady, Sophia Phan, Tanu Vasu, Tash Williams, Teru Morihira, Willa Zheng, and Yu Chieh Chen.